Edited by E.I. Hernández-Jiménez, A.V. Novitskaya

DRY SKIN,
ATOPIC DERMATITIS,
AND PSORIASIS

IN COSMETIC DERMATOLOGY
& SKINCARE PRACTICE

Cosmetics & Medicine
Publishing

Author/Editor:
Elena I. Hernández-Jiménez, *Ph.D.*

Editor:
Anastasia V. Novitskaya, *M.D.* Dermatologist

Contributors:
Vera I. Albanova, *M.D., Ph.D., Prof.* Dermatologist
Natalya G. Kalashnikova, *M.D.* Surgeon, dermatologist, laser therapist
Diana S. Urakova, *M.D., Ph.D.* Dermatologist, laser therapist

DRY SKIN, ATOPIC DERMATITIS, AND PSORIASIS IN COSMETIC DERMATOLOGY AND SKINCARE PRACTICE

The book explores modern skincare and aesthetic methods, providing practical recommendations for effective care aimed specifically for dry skin. It discusses strategies for maintaining remission, alleviating acute symptoms, and addressing aesthetic issues, emphasizing cosmetic approaches that can significantly enhance patients' quality of life.

The book provides a comprehensive analysis of the causes and mechanisms that contribute to the development of dryness. Dry skin is recognized as a distinct clinical condition and one of the main signs of chronic dermatological diseases like atopic dermatitis, and psoriasis. For many years, it was believed that only dermatologists were qualified to treat chronic skin conditions. However, recent research emphasizes that disruption of the epidermal barrier is a key factor in the evolution of atopic dermatitis and psoriasis. Restoring the skin's barrier function is thus crucial in managing dry skin, regardless of the underlying cause. This presents significant opportunities for skincare practitioners to utilize specialized products and procedures to help improve various skin ailments and restore patients' confidence.

In this book, a distinct section is dedicated to each disease, its pathogenesis, and skin characteristics. Subsequent chapters offer insights into the possibilities and limitations of various skincare procedures, aesthetic treatments, and nutritional support. They also provide recommendations for cleansing the skin, choosing basic care products, and evaluating cosmetic ingredients.

Particular attention is given to the skin microbiome and its role in atopic dermatitis and psoriasis, given that maintaining a healthy microbiome, both on the skin and in the gut, has been shown to significantly influence the progression of these diseases and improve the overall skin condition.

This book will serve as a valuable resource for skincare practitioners looking to deepen their knowledge and effectively address the dermatological concerns of their patients. By combining insights from dermatology and cosmetology, it offers innovative approaches that can yield tangible benefits in skincare practice.

ISBN 978-1-970196-46-7 (paperback)
ISBN 978-1-970196-47-4 (hardcover)
ISBN 978-1-970196-48-1 (eBook – Adobe PDF)
ISBN 978-1-970196-49-8 (eBook – ePUB)

Author/Editor

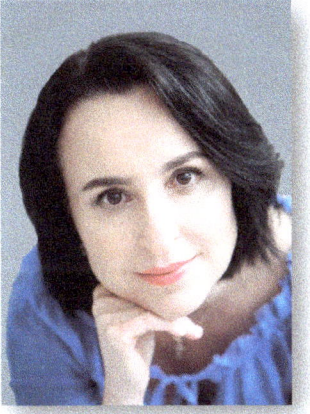

Elena I. Hernández-Jiménez, *Ph.D.*

Biophysicist, scientific journalist

Editor-in-chief of Cosmetics and Medicine Publishing

Chairperson of the Executive Board of the International Society of Applied Corneotherapy (I.A.C.)

Author and co-author of numerous publications in professional magazines, co-author and editor of the book series *Fundamentals of Cosmetic Dermatology & Skincare*, *Cosmetic Dermatology & Skincare Practice*, *Cosmetic Chemistry for Dermatology & Skincare Specialists* and others

Speaker at international conferences, author of training seminars and webinars for professionals in the field of skincare

Professional interests: biology and physiology of the skin, skin permeability, cosmetic chemistry, anti-age medicine, physiotherapy in dermatology and aesthetic medicine, skin analysis and imaging

Table of Contents

PART II
ATOPIC DERMATITIS

List of abbreviations

AAD — American Academy of Dermatology

AD — atopic dermatitis

AHA — alpha-hydroxy acid

AhR — aryl hydrocarbon receptor

ALA — α-linolenic acid

AMP — antimicrobial peptide

AQP3 — aquaporin 3

ASPSG — Asia Scalp Psoriasis Study Group

AU — arbitrary units

BDI — Beck Depression Index

BHA — beta-hydroxy acid

BSA — body surface area

BTA — botulinum toxin type A

CC — clonal complex

CFU — colony forming unit

CGRP — calcitonin gene-related peptide

CNS — central nervous system

DC — dendritic cell

DHA — docosahexaenoic acid

DLQI — Dermatology Life Quality Index

DNA — deoxyribonucleic acid

EASI — Eczema Area and Severity Index

ECM — extracellular matrix

EDC — epidermal differentiation complex

EGF — epithelial growth factor

EPA — eicosapentaenoic acid

Er:YAG — erbium-doped yttrium-aluminum-garnet laser

Er:YSGG — erbium-doped yttrium-scandium-gallium-garnet laser

EVOO — extra-virgin olive oil

FDA — the U.S. Food and Drug Administration

FFA — free fatty acid

FLG — gene encoding filaggrin

FTU — fingertip unit

GAG — glycosaminoglycan

GALT — gut-associated lymphoid tissue

GCS — glucocorticosteroid

HA — hyaluronic acid

HIF-1α — hypoxia-inducible factor 1α

HIFEM — high-intensity focused electromagnetic energy

HIFU — high-intensity focused ultrasound

IBD — inflammatory bowel disease

IFN — interferon

Ig — immunoglobulin

IL — interleukin

ILC2 — type 2 innate immune lymphoid cell

INCI — International Nomenclature of Cosmetic Ingredients

IPL — intensive pulse light

ISAAC — International Study of Asthma and Allergy in Childhood

IU — international units

LED — light-emitting diode

LHA — lipohydroxy acid

MCP-1 — monocyte chemostatic factor 1

MED — minimal erythema dose

MHC — major histocompatibility complex

MMP — matrix metalloproteinase

MUFAs — monounsaturated fatty acids

Nd:YAG/KTP — neodymium-doped yttrium-aluminum-garnet / potassium-titanyl-phosphate laser

NGF — nerve growth factor

NGM — neonatal gut microbiota

NK — natural killer

NMF — natural moisturizing factor

NPY — neuropeptide Y

NSAIDs — non-steroidal anti-inflammatory drugs

PASI — Psoriasis Area and Severity Index

PCA — pyroglutamic acid

PDGF — platelet-derived growth factor

PDL — pulsed dye laser

PHA — polyhydroxy acid

POEM — Patient-Oriented Eczema Measure

PRP — platelet-rich plasma

PSORS — psoriasis susceptibility loci

PUFAs — polyunsaturated fatty acids

RF — radio frequency

ROS — reactive oxygen species

RXR — retinoid X receptor

SASP — senescence-associated secretory program

SCCNFP — The Scientific Committee on Cosmetic Products and Non-food Products Intended for Consumers

SCFA — short-chain fatty acid

SCORAD — Scoring of Atopic Dermatitis

SE — staphylococcal enterotoxin

SMA — spatially modulated ablation

SMAS — superficial muscle-aponeurotic system

SOD — superoxide dismutase

SP — substance P

SPF — sun protection factor

TCA — trichloroacetic acid

TEWL — transepidermal water loss

tGCS — topical glucocorticosteriod

TGF — tumor growth factor

TGF-β — transforming growth factor-β

Th1 — T helper 1 cells

Th2 — T helper 2 cells

TLR — toll-like receptor

TNFα — tumor necrosis factor α

TSLC — thymic stromal lymphopoietin cell

TSST-1 — toxic shock syndrome toxin-1

UCA — urocanic acid

UV — ultraviolet

UVA — ultraviolet type A

UVB — ultraviolet type B

VDR — vitamin D receptor

VEGF — vascular endothelial growth factor

VIP — vasoactive intestinal peptide

Part I

Dry skin

Everyone experiences the discomfort of dry skin during their lifetime. This condition may be temporary, a characteristic feature of the skin, or a symptom of a skin disease. The term "dry skin" encompasses many clinical conditions, each with its causes (Voegeli R., Rawlings A.V., 2023). Depending on the severity of skin dryness, a patient will be bothered by its dull appearance, marked roughness, and flaking, as well as itching, tingling, burning, redness, skin tightness, and usually pain, especially in cases involving facial skin (Voegeli R., Rawlings A.V., 2013).

"Dry skin" primarily means "dry *stratum corneum*." One of the principal differences between the *stratum corneum* and other layers of the epidermis is its relatively low water content — about 15% of dry weight. If the *stratum corneum* lacks water, it becomes stiff, and its altered biomechanical properties can affect the functioning of various skin mechanoreceptors. Most symptoms of dry skin manifest as discomforting sensations that can impair quality of life.

Yet, despite decades of development of moisturizing creams, dry skin remains a serious problem worldwide. While this may seem surprising, the fundamental biochemical features of the *stratum corneum* in different anatomical regions and skin types, as well as the role of age and ethnicity, are still poorly understood.

A finely tuned set of interrelated biochemical and biophysical mechanisms maintains the *stratum corneum*'s water balance. Dry skin develops when one or more of these vital processes malfunction, compromising the skin's ability to retain water during cell differentiation and maturation.

Chapter 1
Dry skin: causes and symptoms

1.1. The *stratum corneum* is the driest tissue in our body

In healthy skin, there is a balance between the amount of water from deeper layers of the epidermis and evaporation from the surface. The degree of *stratum corneum* hydration depends not on the rate at which water passes through it but on the ability of the corneocytes to retain water. As long as the *stratum corneum* can maintain enough moisture for its function, it makes little difference whether 1 ml/cm²/h or 1 µl/cm²/h is evaporated to maintain skin hydration (Scott I.R. et al., 1993).

Well-moisturized skin is soft and smooth, while dry skin is rough, brittle, and cracks easily at creases. For instance, Blank I.H. et al. (1952) found that skin retains its smoothness and softness until the water content is reduced to about 10% of its dry weight. This corresponds to an isolated *stratum corneum*'s relative hydration of about 60%. Below this value, the *stratum corneum* dries out and becomes brittle and dysfunctional. Moreover, the authors demonstrated that water content is more critical for maintaining *stratum corneum*'s elasticity than applying topical oils.

Twenty years later, Wildnauer R.H. et al. (1971) studied *stratum corneum*'s biomechanical properties. They determined that, at a relative humidity of 98%, the *stratum corneum* can stretch in length almost twice before tearing. Under these conditions, the modulus of elasticity (Young's modulus) of *stratum corneum*, which characterizes the ability of the material to resist tension and compression under elastic deformation, is equal to 3 MPa. At a relative humidity of 76%, the *stratum corneum* can stretch by only half, and the modulus of elasticity increases by 20 times (the higher the Young's modulus, the lower the material's elasticity). At 32% moisture content, the *stratum corneum* becomes rigid, and the elastic modulus increases by manifold. Imagine what happens in even drier conditions. Water content and water-holding capacity are key elements in controlling the biomechanics of *stratum corneum*.

Warner R.R. and colleagues (1988) were the first to determine the water concentration profile of the epidermis. Using electron probe analysis and analytical electron microscopy, the authors observed a steep gradient in water content, reaching a plateau in the living epidermis. The living epidermis layers are well-hydrated and contain large quantities of free water. In turn, the *stratum corneum* is the driest tissue in our body and the only skin layer that can function at low hydration levels. This water gradient in the epidermis is responsible for the modulation and regulation of various enzyme cascades involved in the maturation of the *stratum corneum*.

Based on data provided by Warner R.R. and colleagues, it can be estimated that dry body skin requires only 3 ml of bound water for adequate hydration, while dry facial skin requires only 100 µl (Voegeli R. et al., 2013). Why do available moisturizers still fail to effectively address dry skin when such a small amount of water is required, especially considering that water moves through our skin in much larger volumes through sweating and transepidermal water loss (TEWL)?

The degree of skin hydration depends on various structural and physiological parameters, including the composition of the skin barrier, the types and characteristics of the cells involved in barrier function, and internal and external modulating factors.

1.1.1. Role of the epidermal barrier in ensuring optimal skin hydration

The main task of human skin is to form a barrier between the organism's internal environment and the surrounding world. This barrier is two-sided: on the one hand, the skin protects from external influences (chemical compounds, physical and mechanical factors, biological pathogens), and on the other, it prevents physiologically important components (water and electrolytes) from leaving the body, precluding dehydration.

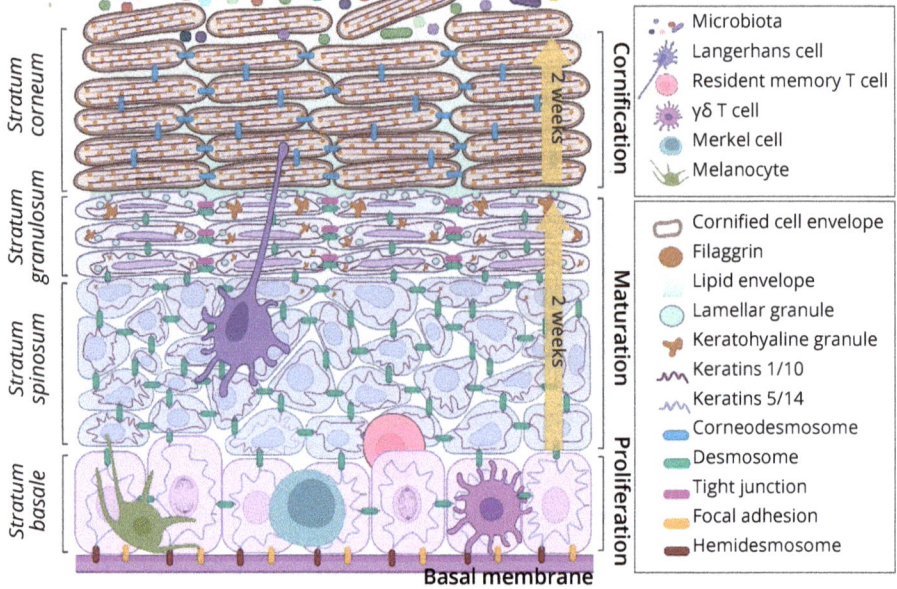

Figure I-1-1. Structure of the epidermis (adapted from Gallegos-Alcalá P. et al., 2021)

Morphological layers of the epidermis

Four layers are distinguished in the epidermis (**Fig. I-1-1**):

1. *Stratum basale*
2. *Stratum spinosum*
3. *Stratum granulosum*
4. *Stratum corneum*

It should be emphasized that these are not anatomical layers of the skin, such as epidermis, dermis, and subcutaneous fatty tissue, which consist of different cells and have various origins, but **morphological layers** — their primary cell is the keratinocyte, which is at different stages of the lifecycle. In this regard, calling them cell layers would be more correct, but the terminology has already been established.

Separation of the morphological layers within the epidermis is associated with the migration and differentiation of keratinocytes. During its life course, which begins with the division of the basal keratinocyte (stem cell) and the detachment of one of the two daughter cells from the basal membrane, the keratinocyte changes externally. Each morphological layer comprises keratinocytes at the same developmental stage and of similar appearance.

Desmosomes and tight junctions between keratinocytes

In contrast to the dermis, where large intercellular spaces separate cells, keratinocytes are packed densely in the epidermis, so water and dissolved substances diffuse through narrow gaps between them. Moreover, protein bridges (desmosomes) and unique structures called tight junctions connect keratinocytes.

Desmosomes are responsible for epidermal density and cell adhesion. They are complex disk-shaped structures with a diameter of several hundred nanometers. Each cell has a circular connective plaque at the junction, from which many intermediate filaments branch out (**Fig. I-1-2**). At the basal plate, keratinocytes are connected by hemidesmosomes. The desmosomes become more pronounced as they extend out of the basal layer. In the *stratum corneum*, they are transformed into **corneodesmosomes**.

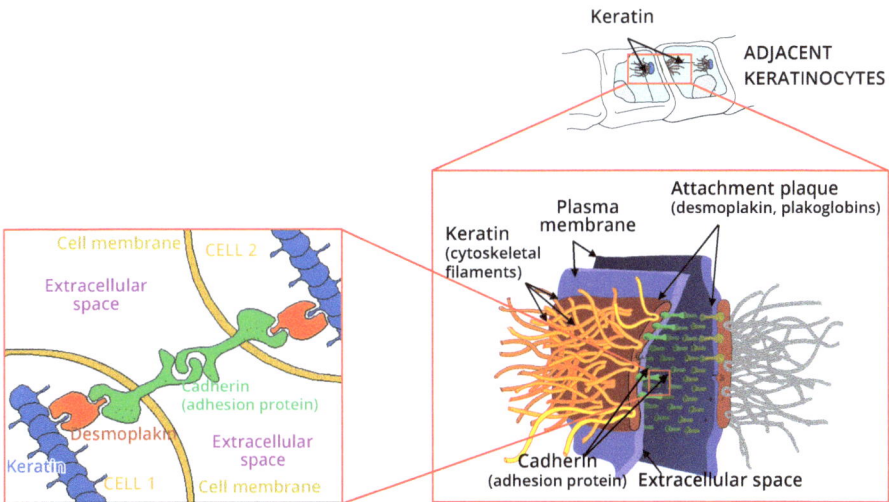

Figure I-1-2. Connection of two keratinocytes by desmosomes (adapted from Wikipedia)

Dense junctions are formed through point connections between the membranes of neighboring cells via transmembrane proteins (claudin-1 and occludin), creating a 0.1–0.5 µm wide belt along the cell's perimeter (usually at its apical pole). As a result, a special kind of lattice or network is formed, which "seals" the intercellular space between the keratinocytes of the granular layer. Owing to its capacity to block the movement of macromolecules and fluids between cells selectively, the network maintains the barrier function of the epidermis and — together with the *stratum corneum* — regulates the transport of substances through it (**Fig. I-1-3**). Recent studies have shown that such contacts help form a reliable barrier already at the granular layer of the epidermis (Yokouchi M., Kubo A., 2018).

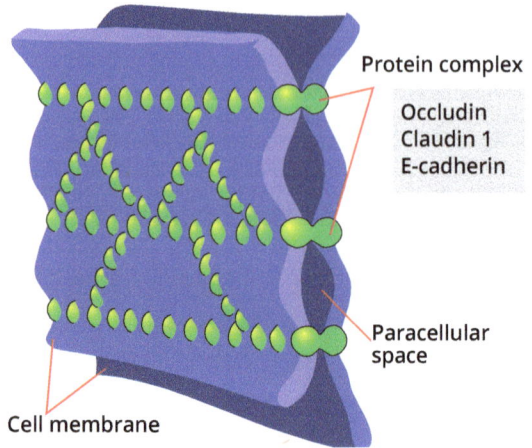

Figure I-1-3. Dense junctions between keratinocyte membranes (adapted from Wikipedia)

Labels: Protein complex — Occludin, Claudin 1, E-cadherin; Paracellular space; Cell membrane

Aquaporins — protein channels in cell membranes that ensure the passage of water — are an essential regulator of skin hydration (Dumas M. et al., 2007). While aquaporins are a common structural component of keratinocyte membranes, they are practically absent from the *stratum corneum*. This ensures the skin is isolated from the environment and water retention is maintained. Aquaporin 3 (AQP3) is most abundant in the skin, which promotes water excretion and glycerol transport within the *stratum corneum* to maintain hydration (Lee Y. et al., 2012). AQP3 has been reported to regulate keratinocyte proliferation, cell migration, and carcinogenesis (Nakahigashi K. et al., 2011). AQP3 expression disorders are associated with skin diseases such as psoriasis and atopic dermatitis (Voss K.E. et al., 2011).

1.1.2. Formation of the *stratum corneum*

As the keratinocytes move toward the surface, they undergo many changes that predetermine the formation of protective structures in the uppermost horny layer. The cells become less flexible, and many different granules form and accumulate in them:

- **Dark granules** contain keratohyalin — the precursor of keratin that will later be formed, as well as profilaggrin, the precursor of filaggrin.
- **Light granules (otherwise known as lamellar bodies or Odland bodies)** are filled with lipids crucial for forming the *stratum corneum*'s permeability barrier and enzymes for processing them.

Keratohyalin and filaggrin of dark granules play a key role in epidermis keratinization and the formation of strong, elastic, protective *stratum corneum*. Keratin, a derivative of keratohyalin, forms filamentous polymers — intermediate filaments in epithelial cells. Filaggrin is needed for intermediate filaments to form a densely ordered network of keratin filaments, providing the *stratum corneum* with mechanical strength. Free filaggrin binds to the intermediate keratin filaments, causing them to aggregate into microfibrils where the intermediate filaments are connected and tightly packed in parallel. This process contributes to the thickening of horny scales.

Filaggrin is further processed by various enzymes (peptidases) in the *stratum corneum*, releasing free amino acids and several metabolites, including pyroglutamic and *trans*-urocanic acids, which are components of natural moisturizing factor (NMF) (**Fig. I-1-4**).

In addition, the NMF complex includes other low-molecular-weight hydrophilic substances such as urea (in concentration up to 10%) and lactic acid (in 5–10% concentration). NMF is located inside the corneocytes, accounting for approximately 10% of their mass and 20–30% of the *stratum corneum* dry weight (Verdier-Sévrain S., Bonté F., 2007). The primary function of NMF is to keep the *stratum corneum* hydrated by absorbing water from the atmosphere due to its components' water solubility and hygroscopicity (Mojumdar E.H., Sparr E., 2021). This process can occur even at 50% relative humidity,

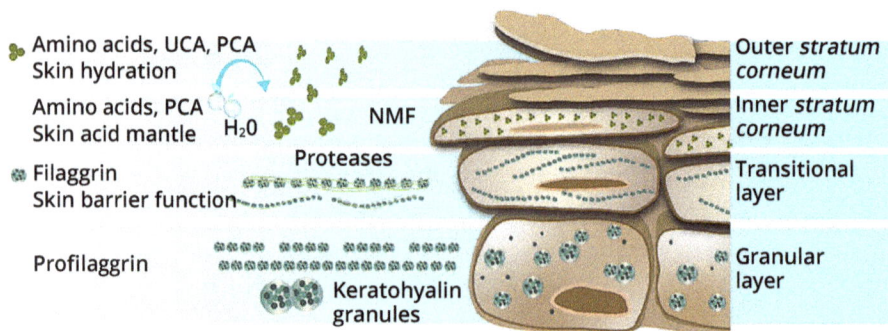

Figure I-1-4. The process of natural moisturizing factor (NMF) production. The precursor protein, profilaggrin, is present in keratinocytes in the granular layer. When cells transform into corneocytes, proteases cleave profilaggrin to filaggrin, which binds keratin filaments together; PCA — pyroglutamic acid, UCA — urocanic acid (adapted from Fowler J., 2012)

allowing corneocytes to maintain adequate hydration under low humidity conditions. The amount of NMF in the *stratum corneum* determines how much water it can retain. Water absorption is so efficient that NMF dissolves in the absorbed water. Its hydrated components (especially the neutral and essential amino acids) form ionic bonds with the keratin fibers, reducing the intermolecular forces between the fibers and thus increasing the elasticity of the *stratum corneum*. Elasticity prevents cracking or flaking due to mechanical stress. In addition, NMF allows the corneocytes to balance the osmotic pressure exerted by the surrounding intercellular "cement." Maintaining a balanced concentration of dissolved substances is essential to prevent excessive water influx, as in the case of skin swelling during prolonged exposure to water or, conversely, loss of water and corneocyte volume reduction (Fowler J., 2012).

Reduced NMF levels are associated with skin dryness, flaking, and cracking (Fowler J., 2012). NMF prevents water loss, protects the skin from colonization by pathogens, and hinders the penetration of toxic substances and allergens. Under ultraviolet (UV) light, *trans*-urocanic acid is transformed into *cis*-urocanic acid, reducing skin sensitivity to UV rays and having an immunomodulatory effect.

Lamellar bodies contain mainly sphingolipids, cholesterol, phospholipids, catabolic enzymes, and antimicrobial peptides. At the border between the granular and the *stratum corneum* layers, lamellar bodies approach the cell membrane, fuse with it, and spill their contents into the extracellular space. Here, lipids undergo enzymatic transformations. As a result, glycerol (known for its moisture-retaining properties) and free fatty acids (FFAs) are formed from phospholipids under the action of phospholipase, and ceramides are formed from sphingolipids, which assemble into lamellar structures and create a lipid barrier (**Fig. I-1-5**) (Feingold K.R., Elias P.M., 2014).

At the border of the granular and *stratum corneum* layers with the keratinocyte, a significant transformation takes place — the cell loses its nucleus, and the living keratinocyte turns into a nucleus-free

SURFACE LIPIDS: TWO FRACTIONS

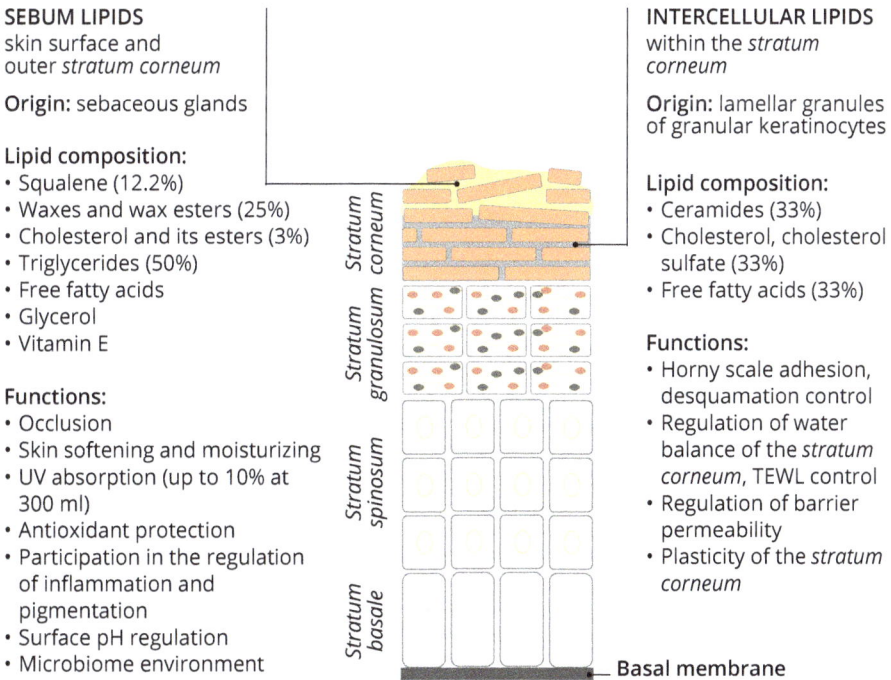

SEBUM LIPIDS
skin surface and
outer *stratum corneum*

Origin: sebaceous glands

Lipid composition:
• Squalene (12.2%)
• Waxes and wax esters (25%)
• Cholesterol and its esters (3%)
• Triglycerides (50%)
• Free fatty acids
• Glycerol
• Vitamin E

Functions:
• Occlusion
• Skin softening and moisturizing
• UV absorption (up to 10% at 300 ml)
• Antioxidant protection
• Participation in the regulation of inflammation and pigmentation
• Surface pH regulation
• Microbiome environment

INTERCELLULAR LIPIDS
within the *stratum corneum*

Origin: lamellar granules of granular keratinocytes

Lipid composition:
• Ceramides (33%)
• Cholesterol, cholesterol sulfate (33%)
• Free fatty acids (33%)

Functions:
• Horny scale adhesion, desquamation control
• Regulation of water balance of the *stratum corneum*, TEWL control
• Regulation of barrier permeability
• Plasticity of the *stratum corneum*

Stratum corneum
Stratum granulosum
Stratum spinosum
Stratum basale
Basal membrane

Figure I-1-5. Lipids of the *stratum corneum* (two fractions): location, source, composition, and functions

High lipid level (hydrophobic)

Rigid corneocytes (mature)

Cornification

Low lipid level

Fragile corneocytes (immature)

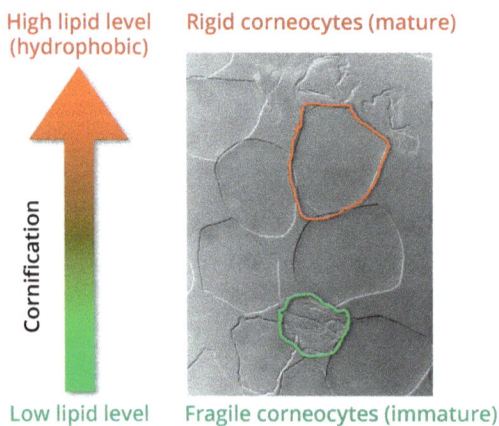

Figure I-1-6. Characteristic features of mature and immature corneocytes (adapted from Voegeli R., Rawlings A.V., 2023)

corneocyte. When initially formed, corneocytes are immature; they are fragile and do not have a good hydrophobic coating. They advance toward the skin surface during keratinization, becoming more hydrophobic and stronger. Fragile or immature cornified cells are smaller and have a rougher surface than rigid or mature cells, characterized by a polygonal shape and a smoother surface (**Fig. I-1-6**).

Corneodesmosomes provide strong intercellular adhesion within the *stratum corneum*, allowing it to resist external mechanical impact, which is crucial for maintaining the barrier function of the epidermis. There is a particular gradient of corneodesmosome density: it is the highest in the lower layers and gradually decreases towards the surface, indicating that the destruction of these structures is essential for the normal *stratum corneum* functioning (Chapman S.J., Walsh A., 1990). The corneodesmosome surplus in the lower layers relative to the upper ones results in the artificial division of the *stratum corneum* into a compact lower layer (*stratum compactum*) and a more superficial loose layer (*stratum disjunctum*), which can be visualized by staining. The skin of the face is characterized by a lower expression or complete absence of the *stratum disjunctum*, which leads to a smaller number of cell layers, smaller corneocyte size, and denser *stratum corneum* compared to other anatomical regions, except palms (Bhawan J. et al., 1992).

Corneocytes are surrounded by a horny envelope consisting of an inner protein envelope and an outer lipid envelope. The lipid monolayer

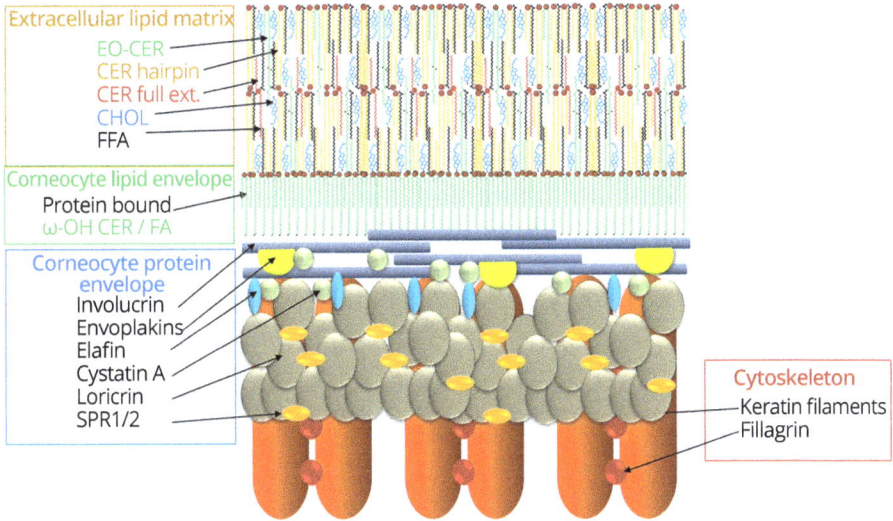

Figure I-1-7. The cornified envelope comprises the intercellular cytoskeleton, the cross-linked, rigid inner protein envelope, and the outer lipid monolayer shell attached to the protein envelope. The lipid monolayer serves as the scaffold for the lamellar organization of the extracellular lipid matrix (adapted from Voegeli R., Rawlings A.V., 2023)

is covalently attached to the protein shell and serves as the basis for the lamellar organization of the extracellular lipid matrix (**Fig. I-1-7**).

Among surface lipids, two fractions are distinguished that differ in origin, composition, and properties:

1. **Lipids of the *stratum corneum*** — located between the horny scales, forming multi-layered lamellar lipid structures (they are usually called the lipid barrier)
2. **Sebum lipids** — part of the hydrolipid (or acid) mantle that covers the skin from the outside in

Lipids of the *stratum corneum*

The composition of lipid layers of the *stratum corneum* differs from the composition of lipid membranes of living epidermal cells. In both cases, amphiphilic lipids — fat molecules having two constituent parts: hydrophilic ("head") and hydrophobic ("tail") — are the main

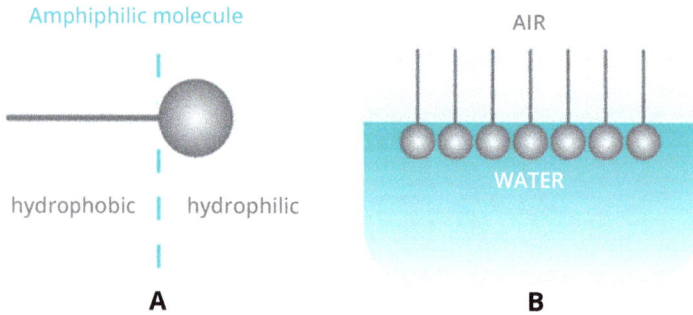

Figure I-1-8. An amphiphilic molecule with a hydrophilic and a hydrophobic part at the interface between air and water

constituents (**Fig. I-1-8**). This structure allows them to self-organize into lipid bilayers. However, while the predominant class of fats in the living layers of the epidermis are phospholipids of cell membranes, in the *stratum corneum*, the dominant positions will be evenly distributed among three types of lipids: **ceramides (CER)**, **cholesterol (CHOL)**, and **free fatty acids (FFAs)**. They are present in equimolar amounts — 1:1:1 (i.e., one molecule of cholesterol and free fatty acid per ceramide molecule) — and the corresponding mass ratios are shown in **Table I-1-1**.

Table I-1-1. Mass ratios of different types of lipids in the *stratum corneum* composition

LIPID SPECIES	W/W, %
Ceramides	40–50
Cholesterol	20–25
Cholesterol sulfate	5–10
Free fatty acids	15–20

The 1:1:1 molar ratio is maximally physiological and provides good barrier functions for the *stratum corneum*. Still, the specific amount of lipids will vary depending on the localization of the skin area and its thickness, as well as the person's age, sex, race, general health, and prevailing climatic conditions (Yang L. et al., 1995).

In addition to these significant lipids, the lipid barrier is also composed of:

- **Cholesterol sulfate** which plays a role in desquamation as a significant inhibitor of serine proteases that degrade corneodesmosomes; it is degraded by steroid sulfatase
- **Free sphingoid bases** formed due to the destruction of ceramides by ceramidases, which have antimicrobial properties and regulate keratinization processes by inhibiting protein kinase C (Feingold K.R., Elias P.M., 2014)

Thus, its main components' qualitative composition and balanced ratio are essential to ensuring the *stratum corneum*'s structural and barrier integrity.

The lipid layers of the *stratum corneum* are parallel and separated by a thin aqueous layer through which water moves toward the surface and evaporates. This process is called **transepidermal water loss (TEWL)**. Water movement is facilitated when the lipid barrier structure is disrupted and water evaporates more quickly.

Sebum — a sebaceous gland secretion composed of triglycerides, wax esters, squalene, and some free fatty acids (**Table I-1-2**) — provides additional protection (see **Fig. I-1-5**). The sebum level depends on the anatomical region (**Fig. I-1-9**).

Table I-1-2. Mass ratios of different types of lipids in the hydrolipid mantle composition

LIPID SPECIES	W/W, %
Triglycerides	42
Free fatty acids	15
Wax esters	25
Squalene	15
Cholesterol esters	2
Cholesterol	1
Carotenoids, vitamin E, etc.	<1

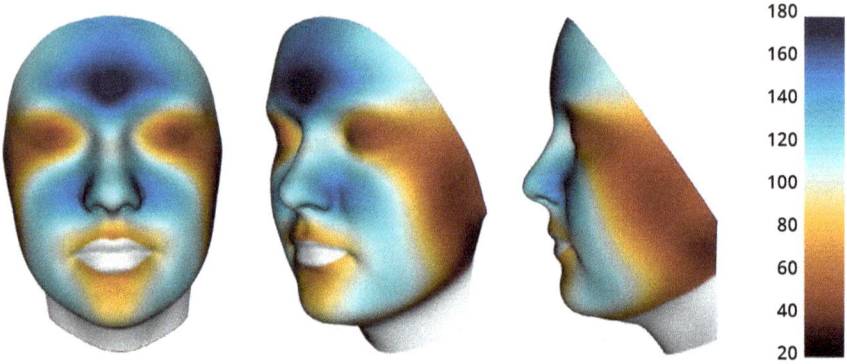

Figure I-1-9. Changes in sebum levels in different areas of the face according to a study involving 12 women (mean age 44 years) (adapted from Voegeli R. et al., 2019)

Sebum can enhance skin barrier function by minimizing water loss, providing optimal thermoregulation and protection against pathogens, and exhibiting photoprotective properties (**Fig. I-1-10**). Sebum also influences the composition of the skin microbiome because it

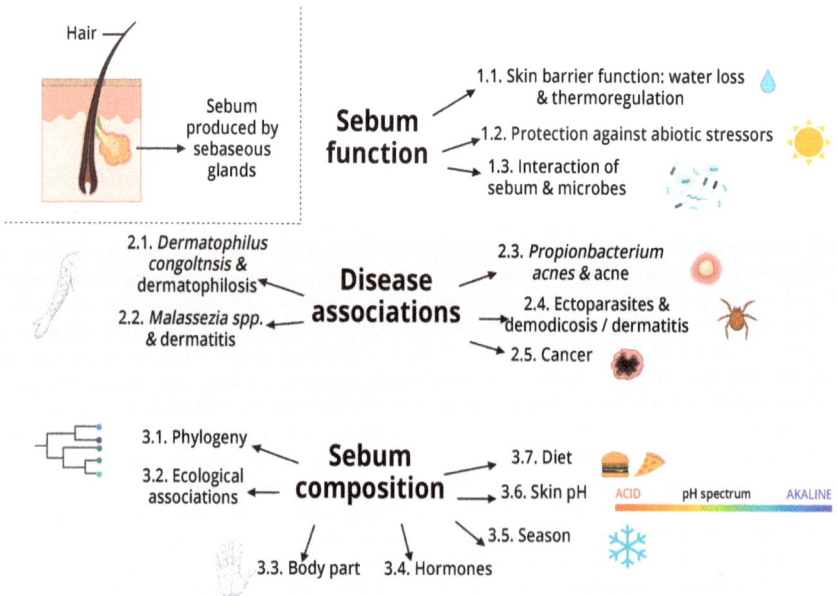

Figure I-1-10. Role of sebaceous glands in maintaining skin health (adapted from Vanderwolf K. et al., 2023)

serves as a potential source of nutrients and has antimicrobial properties (Vanderwolf K. et al., 2023). On the skin surface, sebum mixes with sweat gland secretion and transepidermal water — this is how the **hydrolipidic mantle** is formed. Sebum softens its top layer, exerts an antimicrobial effect, and reduces moisture loss. Water evaporation is inhibited by smoothing the horny scales as well as by the glycerin present in the sebum. At the same time, oxygen and carbon dioxide pass through the hydrolipidic mantle entirely freely.

1.1.3. Desquamation

Proteolytic enzymes destroy the corneodesmosomes connecting the corneocytes, causing them to leave the skin surface — this process is called **desquamation**.

Desquamation can only occur after the extracellular portion of the corneodesmosomes has been hydrolyzed by proteases (mainly kallikreins) and cathepsins and deglycosylated by heparinase and other glycosidases (**Fig. I-1-11**). The enzymes are under the control of endogenous inhibitors such as LEKTI, SLPI, or elafin (Rawlings A.V.,

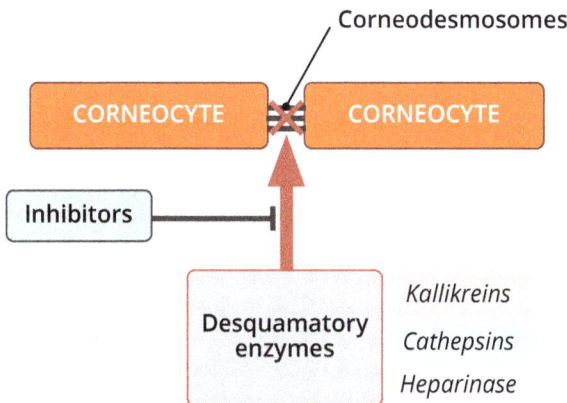

Figure I-1-11. Corneocyte desquamation can only occur after corneodesmosomes are hydrolyzed by specific proteases that are kept under control by inhibitors (adapted from Voegeli R., Rawlings A.V., 2023)

Voegeli R., 2013). Under conditions characterized by constant water deficit, the desquamation of horny scales is impaired, affecting the condition of the entire epidermis. Therefore, the optimal balance between proliferation and desquamation is one of the most critical factors in skin barrier formation.

Data on the structural components of the epidermal barrier and their functions are summarized in **Table I-1-3**.

Table I-1-3. Major components of the epidermal barrier and their functions

COMPONENT	LOCALIZATION	FUNCTION
Corneocyte	*Stratum corneum*	Strength, stiffness, and impermeability of the *stratum corneum*
Corneodesmosomes	Between the corneocytes	Ensuring the integrity of the *stratum corneum*
Granular keratinocytes	Boundary between the *stratum granulosum* and the *stratum corneum*	Source of filaggrin and other NMF precursors, lipid barrier lipids, and the *stratum corneum* enzymes
Lipid barrier	Lamellar lipid layers of the *stratum corneum*	Regulation of diffusion of substances through the *stratum corneum*, including water
Lamellar bodies (Odland bodies)	Boundary between the *stratum granulosum* and the *stratum corneum*	Source of lipid precursors that make up the lipid barrier
Stratum corneum enzymes	Inside the lamellar bodies, the *stratum corneum*	Intercellular matrix lipid synthesis, desquamation of corneocytes
Natural Moisturizing Factor (NMF)	Corneocytes, intercellular space within the *stratum corneum*	Water retention in the *stratum corneum*
pH gradient, Ca^{2+} gradient	*Stratum corneum*	Control of keratinization, secretion of lipid barrier lipid precursors, and the *stratum corneum* enzyme activity

So, what structural features of the epidermal barrier allow the *stratum corneum* to maintain an optimal degree of hydration?

1. **Tight junctions and desmosomes.** Keratinocytes are located close to each other and are separated only by narrow gaps. Because tight junctions and desmosomes bind to keratinocytes, selective blocking of the movement of macromolecules and fluids between cells is achieved. The density of desmosomes gradually decreases toward the surface, allowing water to be retained in the deeper epidermis layers, thereby facilitating the desquamation process.

2. **Aquaporins** in the membranes of keratinocytes are protein channels that allow water to pass in and out of a living cell. Corneocytes (dead cells) do not have aquaporins.

3. **Natural Moisturizing Factor (NMF)** is a complex of small hygroscopic molecules (free amino acids, urea, lactic acid, sodium pyroglutamate) in and around the corneocytes. It binds to and retains water in the *stratum corneum*.

4. **The lipid barrier** controls water evaporation, maintains the *stratum corneum* hydration level, and prevents foreign substances from entering the body.

5. **Sebum** acts as a natural occlusive moisturizer. By forming a film on the skin surface and smoothing the horny scales, it prevents water loss.

6. **Keratin** is a large protein aggregate that fills corneocytes. It is insoluble, but like all proteins, it swells in water and firmly binds water molecules through electrostatic bonds.

When one or more water-retaining structures are impaired (deficiency, structural changes), the water level in the *stratum corneum* decreases. All these elements of the epidermal barrier also serve as therapeutic targets for the correction of dry skin.

1.1.4. Skin microbiome and the barrier function

The skin functions closely with the microorganisms living on its surface — the skin microbiome (**Fig. I-1-12**).

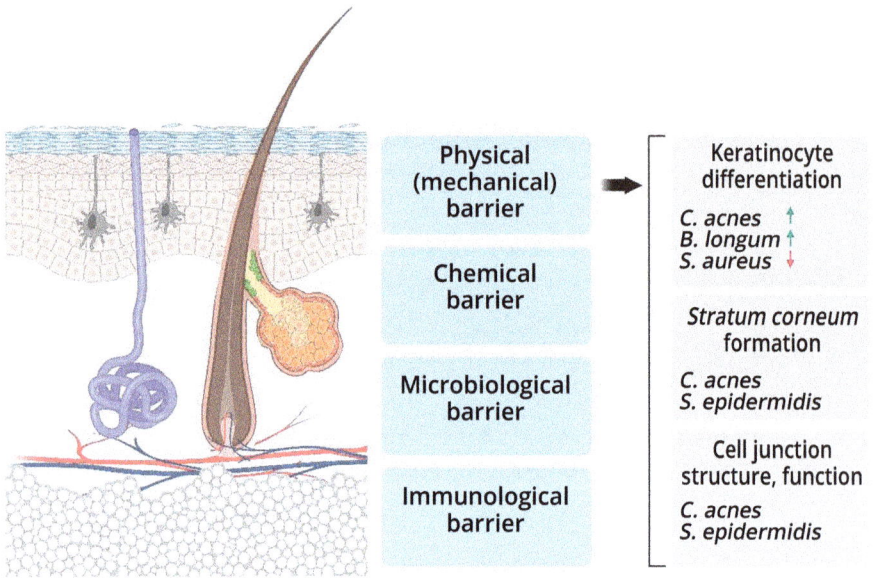

Figure I-1-12. Human skin forms a complex protective barrier. The skin microbiome influences various properties of this complex interface, up to and including functionally mature tissue. The figure shows bacterial strains with proven effects on specific components of the physical barrier. The green arrow indicates positive, and the red arrow indicates adverse effects (adapted from Szabó K. et al., 2023)

Our skin is second only to the intestine in bacterial density, with approximately 10^4–10^6 cells per 1 cm^2 belonging to more than 200 species. The skin is inhabited by representatives of 18 phylogenetic groups, among which four are dominant: *Actinobacteria* (51.8%), *Firmicutes* (24.4%), *Proteobacteria* (16.5%), and *Bacteroidetes* (6.3%) (Cundell A.M., 2018).

One of the key roles of the skin microbiome is to maintain homeostasis by providing nutrients (synthesis of vitamins and amino acids), suppressing the growth of pathogens, "training" the immune system to distinguish between commensal and pathogenic microorganisms, and regulating epidermal differentiation (**Fig. I-1-13**) (Smythe P., Wilkinson H.N., 2023).

Areas with many sebaceous glands (e.g., trunk, back, and face) are highly acidic due to the abundance of free fatty acids. These areas are

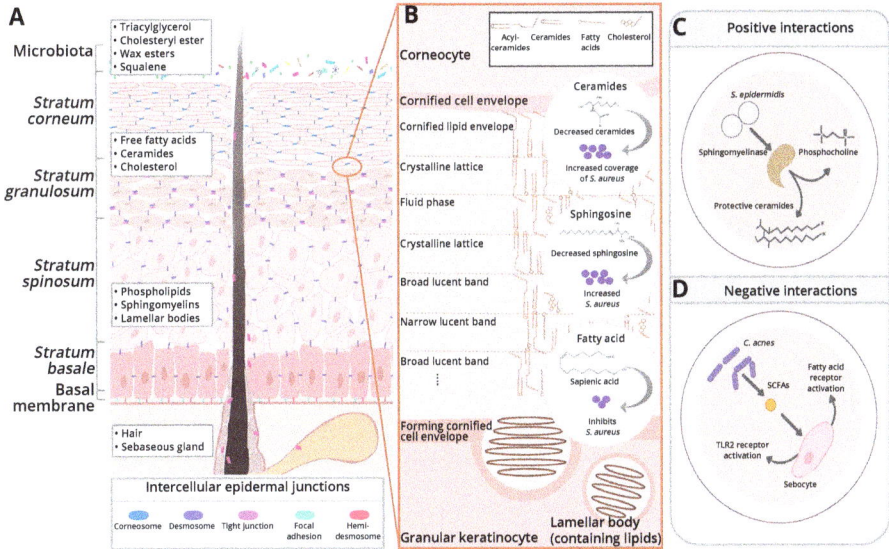

Figure I-1-13. The skin microbiome has a modulating effect on the level and composition of skin lipids (adapted from Smythe P., Wilkinson H.N., 2023)

The epidermis consists of several layers of phenotypically distinct keratinocytes at different stages of differentiation: A — keratinocytes in each tier have different adhesion structures responsible for maintaining skin integrity. Epidermal lipids are present in the differentiating layers of the epidermis, and sebaceous glands secrete sebum lipids; B — molecular arrangement of the major lipids of the *stratum corneum* and the influence of these lipids on *Staphylococcus aureus* colonization; C — skin surface-dwelling microorganisms also produce metabolites involved in lipid cleavage, which makes products that contribute to barrier homeostasis (e.g., sphingomyelinase produced by *Staphylococcus epidermidis*); D — under pathological conditions, these interactions can negatively affect skin physiology (e.g., *Cutibacterium acnes* increases inflammation). SCFAs — short-chain fatty acids

predominantly inhabited by bacteria such as *Cutibacterium*, which can metabolize sebum and tolerate low pH levels.

Anatomical areas characterized by high skin moisture (e.g., elbow fossa, inguinal crease, and hamstring) are sites with higher temperatures and degree of hydration, as well as multiple hair follicles and sweat glands. Such a moist environment is rich in nutrients (including salts, sterols, esters, and lipids), which promote skin colonization by *Staphylococcus* and *Corynebacterium* (Grice E.A. et al., 2009). Whereas *Corynebacteria* dominate warm and moist environments, *Staphylococci* prefer moist, salt-rich sites like sweat glands. Although the microbiome of moist skin remains relatively stable, its abundance and

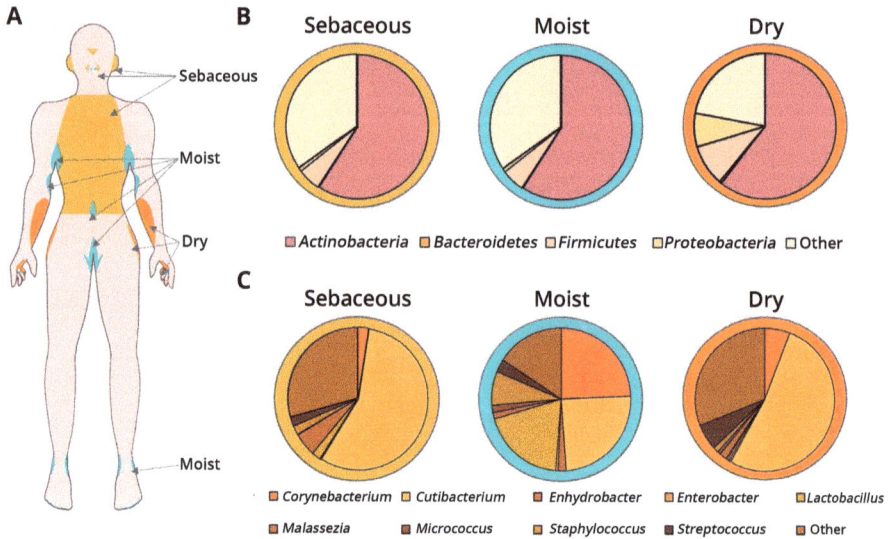

Figure I-1-14. Microenvironmental conditions determine the skin microbiome composition (adapted from Smythe P., Wilkinson H.N., 2023)

Depending on physiologic characteristics, skin is categorized into oily, moist, and dry skin (A). The species composition of the microbiome is influenced by skin pH, temperature, sebum content, and moisture level (B)

species composition vary from person to person. In contrast, dry sites (e.g., the inner surface of the forearm and the little finger area) are characterized by instability and diversity of microbiome composition (**Fig. I-1-14**) (Oh J. et al., 2016).

Russo E. et al. (2023) investigated the peculiarities of microbiome species composition depending on skin type and age. The authors determined the skin type (dry, normal) of 15 healthy women living in the same area and compared the species composition of their respective microbiomes.

Firmicutes species, the class *Clostridia*, and the species *Negativicoccus* and *Peptoniphylus* were significantly more abundant in samples from participants with normal skin than those with dry skin (**Fig. I-1-15**). In contrast, the *Alphaproteobacteria* and *Spirochaetae* were substantially more abundant in dry skin than in normal skin. The authors noted a higher alpha diversity* of the microbiome of dry skin. Although the reported

---

* Alpha diversity is the diversity of microbial species within the gut microbiome of the same individual.

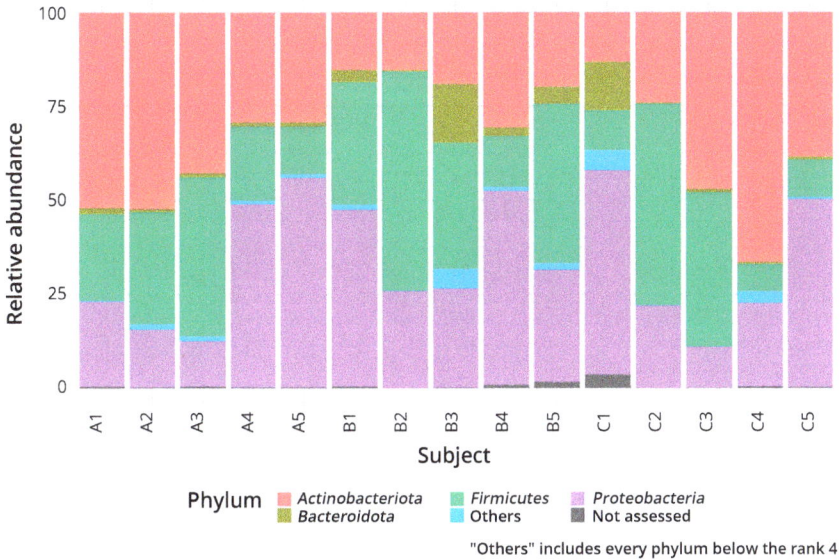

Figure I-1-15. Taxonomic composition of facial skin samples of participants in the dry and normal skin groups. The histogram shows the relative abundance of the four most common bacterial strains (adapted from Russo E. et al., 2023)

results were based on a small sample, they confirmed the influence of hydration level on the microbiome's species composition.

In earlier studies, it has been shown that dry skin and aged skin exhibit higher microbiome alpha diversity. This may indicate an epidermal barrier disruption in these conditions (Kim J.H. et al., 2021).

Skin is a habitat and nutrient source for microorganisms (Harris-Tryon T.A., Grice E.A., 2022). Skin cells recognize the types of microorganisms and obtain information about the current state of the microbiome by direct contact and by sensing microbial molecules (e.g., metabolites, enzymes, and toxins). In turn, microorganisms exert modulatory effects on the chemical and immunologic components of the skin barrier, including keratinocyte differentiation, *stratum corneum* formation, and regulation of intercellular contacts (**Table I-1-4**).

Thus, a healthy microbiome is one of the guarantors of the normal functioning of the epidermal barrier and, consequently, of maintaining optimal skin moisturization.

Table I-1-4. Effect of the microbiome on different components of the epidermal barrier (Szabó K. et al., 2023)

PROCESSES UNDERLYING THE BARRIER FUNCTION	PUTATIVE EFFECTS OF THE MICROBIOME
Keratinocyte differentiation	• Participation in early, neonatal adaptation • Regulation of keratinocyte differentiation by influencing the expression of epidermal differentiation complex (EDC) genes (Uberoi A. et al., 2021)
Formation of the *stratum corneum*	Modulation of lipid barrier and sebum composition (Zheng Y. et al., 2022)
Intercellular junctions	Influencing the structure of dense junctions through changes in the expression of its components (Bolla B.S. et al., 2020)

Since the microbiome significantly impacts the structural and functional state of the epidermal barrier, it can be used as a therapeutic target to improve the skin barrier properties.

1.2. Internal and external factors affecting skin hydration

1.2.1. Ethnicity

Genetics is one of the most important factors determining an organism's structural and functional characteristics. Voegeli R. and colleagues (2019) were among the first to raise the topic of the influence of ethnicity on the degree of skin hydration. Their study sample included 16 young women (mean age 21.8 years) without visual signs of photoaging: four belonged to the African (phototypes V–VI), four to the Caucasoid (phototypes II–III), four to the Chinese (phototypes II–III) and four to the Indian ethnic group (phototypes III–IV) (Voegeli R. et al., 2019).

The authors found significant interethnic differences in facial skin hydration, barrier function, and skin surface pH. Total skin hydration was the highest in participants of the African ethnic group, followed by Indians, Caucasians, and Chinese. In all groups, the nasolabial area and cheeks were characterized by the lowest hydration values and the eye area by the highest (**Fig. I-1-16**). TEWL scores were the highest among Indians, followed by Chinese, Africans, and Caucasians. The lowest TEWL scores were found in the middle and lower cheeks and jaw area, and the highest scores were found around the eyes, in the nasolabial fold, and in the palpebral groove. The discrepancy between the degree of

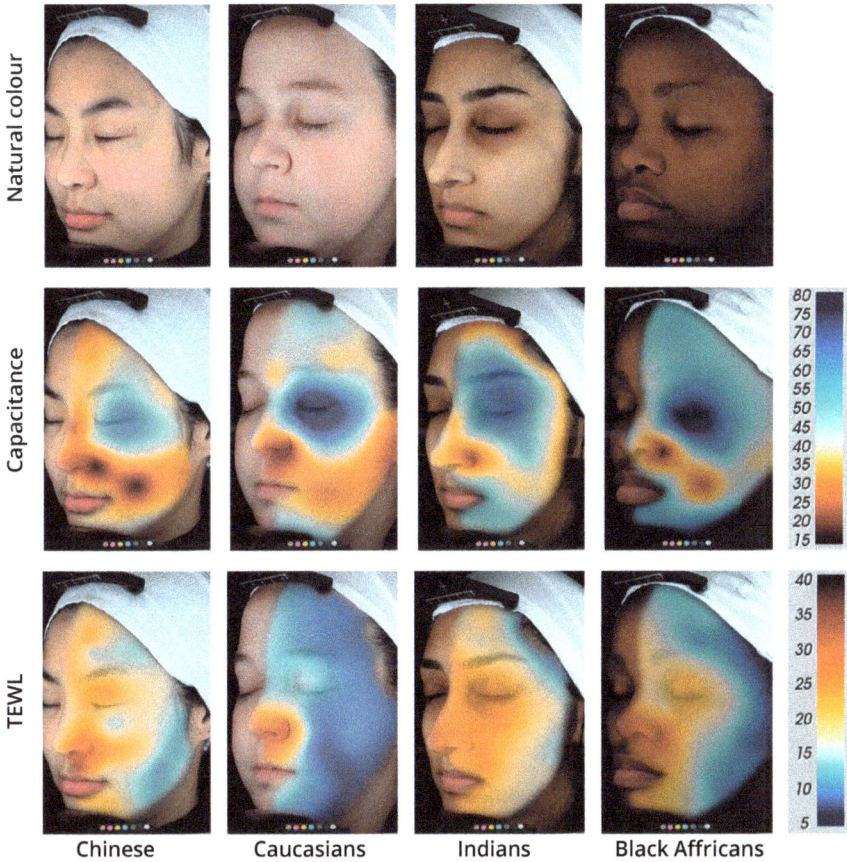

Figure I-1-16. Color schemes characterizing transepidermal water loss (TEWL) and skin hydration in different ethnic groups (from left to right: Chinese, Caucasian, Indian, African). The color code for corneometer values (15–80 AU) and TEWL (5–40 g m^{-2}/h) are shown on the color scales on the right (blue — healthy skin, red — epidermal barrier dysfunction) (adapted from Voegeli R. et al., 2019)

skin hydration and TEWL is evident. Thus, although dark skin was more hydrated, it was also characterized by high TEWL, indicating a weaker protective barrier.

On the other hand, there was no apparent relationship between skin hydration scores (TEWL, degree of hydration) and pH, or epidermal barrier health and degree of skin pigmentation, although more pronounced barrier properties in skin with darker phototypes were previously noted by Young M.M. et al. (2019).

1.2.2. Aging

Research shows that skin moisturization decreases with age, but the mechanisms underlying this process are not fully understood (Nomoto T., Iizaka S., 2020).

In the *stratum corneum*, water is mainly present in the corneocytes and is bound by NMF, while smaller amounts are retained by the polar lipid heads of intercellular layers (Schleusener J. et al., 2021). As the skin ages, NMF content decreases due to insufficient profilaggrin synthesis and impaired barrier function (Rawlings A.V., Harding C.R., 2004).

The age-related decrease in barrier lipid levels, especially ceramides, significantly weakens the epidermal barrier. The aging process also decreases hyaluronic acid content in the dermis. Since hyaluronic acid binds water molecules, its age-related deficiency negatively affects skin hydration (Papakonstantinou E. et al., 2012). Hyaluronic acid's important role in maintaining skin hydration makes it one of the main therapeutic targets in anti-aging medicine (Göllner I. et al., 2017).

1.2.3. Biological rhythms

Biochemical and physiological processess in our organism are subordinated to a certain rhythm, which is one way of adapting to periodically changing environmental conditions. Circadian rhythms are cyclic fluctuations in the intensity of various biological processes associated with the changes in natural light due to the transition from day to night. Circadian rhythms are usually close to 24 hours (Marcheva B. et al., 2013). There are also ultradian rhythms with periods shorter than a day (from minutes to 10–12 hours) (Van Cauter E., 1990).

A central regulator dictates circadian rhythms in the suprachiasmatic nucleus of the anterior hypothalamus. Rhythmic changes in biochemical and physiological processes are realized through the transcription and translation of various circadian clock genes and proteins (Buhr E.D., Takahashi J.S., 2013). Circadian genes modulate the activity of many different types of skin cells and subordinate them to specific biological rhythms (Firooz A. et al., 2016). Two circadian genes (*CLOCK* and *Per1*) are expressed in keratinocytes, melanocytes, and dermal fibroblasts (Zanello S.B. et al., 2000). *CLOCK* has been found to affect AQP3-encoding genes and thus plays a role in skin hydration: the higher the AQP3 expression is, the greater the TEWL and lower the hydration are, and vice versa (Matsunaga N. et al., 2014). Keratinocyte proliferation, sebum secretion, pH, blood flow intensity, and skin temperature are also subject to circadian fluctuations (Lyons A.B. et al., 2019).

In their study involving 16 healthy men and women, Yosipovitch G. et al. (1998) found specific changes in TEWL and the degree of *stratum corneum* hydration. TEWL was measured at two-hour intervals for 24 hours. Time-dependent TEWL dynamics were characteristic of the skin of the forearm, forehead, upper back, and tibia, with TEWL significantly increasing in the evening at all sites and being the lowest in the morning (Yosipovitch G. et al., 1998).

1.2.4. Environment

The main environmental factors contributing to reduced skin hydration are UVB exposure, low temperatures, and low humidity (Camilion J.V. et al., 2022). Low humidity and UV radiation lessen the ability of hydrolytic enzymes to cleave filaggrin to NMF, resulting in a dry skin surface (Biniek K. et al., 2012). In addition, UVB overexposure leads to increased TEWL due to epidermal barrier damage, disrupting cellular cohesion and the mechanical integrity of intercellular lipids and corneodesmosomes (Kwon T.R. et al., 2016).

Seasonal climatic changes also affect skin moisturization. According to the data published by Rogers J. et al. (1996), the lipid levels in the *stratum corneum* decrease in winter relative to the spring and summer periods. The authors recorded a 20% decrease in ceramide 1 linoleate levels in the skin of the lower extremities. They suggested that this decrease in lipid content affects skin hydration, increasing the risk of xerosis and impaired barrier function, especially during winter. These results indicate that linoleic acid esters can be a potential therapeutic agent for enhancing the skin barrier function (Kwon T.R. et al., 2016).

High ambient temperature causes excessive sweating, increasing hydration and TEWL (Kim S. et al., 2019). Song E.J. et al. (2015) investigated the number of skin pores functioning in summer compared to winter. They found that there were more active pores in summer. Based on these findings, they concluded that TEWL and hydration vary depending on the season and anatomical region.

The degree of hydration affects the epidermis structure, barrier permeability, and skin homeostasis. According to Denda M. et al. (1998), low humidity increases epidermal DNA synthesis in normal mouse epidermis. Low humidity stimulates a barrier breakdown response in the form of epidermal hyperplasia. Staying in a dry environment for 48 hours leads to mast cell hypertrophy, degranulation, and inflammation, which may eventually culminate in barrier damage. Environmental humidity changes also increase keratinocyte proliferation and inflammatory marker production. Animals maintained in a dry environment for two weeks showed a decrease in TEWL of nearly 30%, an increase in epidermal thickness, and an increase in the dry horny mass relative to animals kept in a humid climate. The increase in the *stratum corneum* thickness is an adaptive response aimed at reducing TEWL and retaining water in the skin (Ashida Y., Denda M., 2003; Katagiri C. et al., 2003).

1.3. Dehydrated skin: a problem with the dermal matrix

"Dry skin" and "dehydrated skin" conditions are fundamentally different. The former is caused by impaired barrier properties at the *stratum corneum* level, whereas the latter is associated with a water deficit due to changes in the extracellular matrix of the dermis. The main clinical symptom of dehydrated skin is reduced turgor — such skin looks flabby, as if slightly chewed. It may have a few wrinkles, but those present are more prolonged and profound. Often, dehydrated skin takes on a yellowish tint due to microcirculation problems.

The most common causes of dehydrated skin include decreased glycosaminoglycan levels in the extracellular matrix, fibrosis, and accumulation of glycation products.

It should be noted that dry skin may have good turgor, and dehydrated skin may have good barrier properties. In some conditions, the skin has symptoms of both dryness and dehydration. For example, this combination can be observed in photodamaged skin owing to the adverse effects of UV rays on different skin layers and structures.

In dehydrated skin, cosmetic products are of little benefit as they are intended to address the superficial changes at the *stratum corneum* level. Thus, they cannot have a noticeable effect on the dermal layer. Here, we need more "deep"-acting methods like mesotherapy (multiple intradermal injections of bioactive substances in a solution). With the help of a needle, bypassing all natural barriers, it is possible to deliver the necessary substances to the dermal layer, activating the regenerative processes aimed at the structural reorganization of the extracellular matrix. The microtrauma caused by puncturing the skin will be an additional stimulus for recovery.

Unlike cosmetic surface-level moisturizing, which is felt immediately, mesotherapeutic correction of dehydrated skin condition is cumulative. Its effect will be noticeable only after some time because it requires specific structural changes, which occur gradually.

Device-based fractional technologies partially solve the problem of skin dehydration. These methods rely on microtrauma to trigger structural rearrangements in the skin tissue, ideally restoring the matrix and its water-regulating and water-retaining mechanisms.

When working with dry skin, attention should be paid to microcirculation, as it is responsible for water inflow and outflow. Therefore, it is advisable to include special lymphatic drainage massage (microcurrent therapy, manual techniques) in the correction program.

The goal of cosmetic treatment is to normalize the skin water content. Still, the methods of correcting water balance and hydration will differ dramatically depending on the level of exposure and the nature of the structural rearrangements that have led to water deficiency.

Chapter 2
Dry skin hygiene

When caring for dry skin, special attention should be paid to its cleansing, which should be as gentle as possible because we are dealing with skin with a weakened barrier function (Okamoto N. et al., 2017). As no damage to the weak barrier structures should occur during short contact with the skin, a cleanser for dry skin should be chosen as carefully as preparations for moisturizing and care.

2.1. Natural soap

Natural soap's high alkalinity significantly disadvantages the skin barrier. After washing with an alkaline solution, the pH on the skin surface rises, and it takes an average of two hours to restore it to a physiological "acidic" level.

In addition, soap's salt ions can "wash out" NMF components from the *stratum corneum*, and fatty acids can clog pores (especially if the skin is prone to comedone formation). Therefore, it is desirable to reduce the soap solution's contact time with the skin and wash it off as soon as possible with plenty of water. If removing all the dirt at once is impossible, it is better to soap the skin again rather than increase the exposure time.

Frequent use of natural soap can harm the skin. If the skin is exposed to soap before it has time to restore its barrier structures, it can cause irritation and dryness. The risk of adverse reactions is exceptionally high in skin with a weakened barrier (e.g., because of a skin disease such as dermatitis, psoriasis, etc.) and hypersensitivity. Natural soaps must be avoided and replaced with synthetic counterparts (syndets) or emulsion-based or anhydrous cleansers.

2.2. Synthetic soaps (syndets)

Syndets are chemically synthesized from fats, petroleum/oil-based products, or oil-based products (oleochemicals) and alkali compounds through a combination of chemical processes other than saponification, namely sulfonation (the process of attaching a sulfonic acid functional group, $-SO_3H$), ethoxylation (the process of attaching ethylene oxide, C_2H_4O), and esterification (whereby carboxylic acids react with alcohols to form esters). Therefore, syndets usually consist of a mixture of synthetic compounds such as fatty acid isethionates or esters of sulfosuccinic acid (e.g., alkyl sulfates and alkyl sulfosuccinates).

In people with dry skin, including those suffering from eczema, traditional soaps with their characteristically high pH can aggravate the condition, resulting in a loss of intracellular lipids and red, rough, and flaky skin. This damage can affect the nerve endings of the dermis (a hallmark of sensitive skin), resulting in itching, burning, and pain. Disruption of the skin barrier can also promote the entry of allergens and increased multiplication of bacteria such as *S. aureus*. Regarding cleansing, the recommendations remain similar: use mildly acidic, pH-regulated syndets to reduce the impact of infectious organisms, irritants, or allergens and minimize irritation and itching.

Unfortunately, even syndets with favorable mildness can potentially remove key skin components, compromise the integrity and functionality of the *stratum corneum*, and inevitably lead to some weakening of the skin barrier, sensitization, and irritation. Thus, skin should be cleansed carefully, as careless use of cleansing products, especially harsh alkaline soaps, will undoubtedly cause adverse skin reactions. The most appropriate cleansers, such as syndets, should be mild while maintaining a fine balance between cleansing the skin and preserving its homeostatic properties. Additionally, they should cause little or no irritation, disruption, or damage to its physiological parameters, including hydration, the state of the acid mantle, and the overall barrier function.

The ability to adjust the pH of the finished product is a considerable advantage of syndets over natural soaps, making them well-suited for dry, damaged, and/or sensitive skin. In addition, the surfactants in modern syndets act more gently on the skin than those found in natural soaps. Conversely, additives included in soaps (natural or synthetic) can cause unwanted skin reactions. For this reason, it is better to choose products with minimal additive content (at least without colorants and fragrances) for cleansing delicate, sensitive, and/or damaged skin.

2.3. Oil-free cleansing agents

This category includes skin **cleansers** that do not contain oily components (**lipid-free cleansers**), such as shower gels and cleansing solutions (toners). They contain water, glycerin, cetyl alcohol, sterol alcohol, sodium lauryl sulfate, and (sometimes) propylene glycol.

The product is applied to dry or damp skin, whipped up to foam by fingertips (or by a washcloth/sponge for shower gel), and then rinsed with plenty of water. As the foam dissolves and emulsifies fatty deposits and dirt on the skin surface, this gentle cleanser is especially recommended for people with photodamaged skin. However, propylene glycol use can lead to a feeling of tightness and is not recommended for those with very dry skin. In addition, sodium lauryl sulfate, which facilitates foam formation, is an emulsifier with increased irritant potential and should not be applied to the skin with a severely damaged barrier.

2.4. Cleansing emulsions

Emulsion-based products such as cold cream (a thick emulsion) and milk (a liquid emulsion) can cleanse the skin on the face and body. Emulsions are composed of three parts: water, oils, and emulsifiers. By their chemical nature, emulsifiers are surfactants; emulsions are used not to form a foam but to prevent the water and oil phases from separating.

Cold cream is an emulsion with high water content that cools the skin due to water evaporation. The cooling effect also depends on oils and the type of emulsion. It can be water-in-oil or oil-in-water, but it must be thin. In most cold creams, large amounts of water are emulsified by adding borax (sodium decahydrate tetraborate) or mucilaginous substances; for the same purpose, lanolin is introduced in the oil phase of the emulsion. Due to the abundance of water, cold cream quickly spoils. To extend its shelf-life, glycerin can replace water, but such a preparation is no longer a cold cream. On the other hand, stable cold cream can be obtained as a mixture of equal parts of lanolin, almond oil, and water (the amount of water can be increased) with fragrances (e.g., rose oil). In modern preparations, the oil phase can be made from mineral oil, petroleum jelly, and waxes (beeswax, vegetable, synthetic).

When the cream is applied to the skin, part of the fatty components penetrates the intercellular spaces of the *stratum corneum*, and part remains on the surface, softening the skin and moisturizing it due to occlusion (transepidermal evaporation of water is inhibited, and water is concentrated within the *stratum corneum*). At the same time, the water included in the preparation evaporates quickly, making the skin feel cold. For this reason, cold creams are very popular among patients with dry and irritated skin.

Cleansing milk is a light oil-in-water emulsion often used to remove makeup and cleanse delicate facial zones, including areas around the eyes and lips. It is also suitable for people with dry skin. The preparation is applied directly to the skin and is lightly massaged with fingertips or placed on a cotton pad, which is wiped over the skin. The treated area is then rinsed with water or thoroughly wiped with a clean cotton disk soaked in water.

Chapter 3
Fundamentals of topical moisturization

When one or more water-holding structures are disrupted (e.g., due to deficiencies or structural changes), the water level in the horny layer declines. It is logical to assume that the choice of moisturizing strategy will depend on where the failure occurred. Determining the cause by eye can be challenging because dry skin symptoms are independent of the underlying cause. This is where instrumental functional diagnostics methods come to the rescue.

To assess the functional state of the skin, the following methods can be used, depending on the focus of the analysis:

- Cutometry (skin elasticity)
- Ballistometry (viscoelastic properties)
- Reviscometry (anisotropy, i.e., orientation of collagen fibers, which becomes less pronounced with age and pathology)

Functional analysis can be supplemented by structural analysis, allowing visualization of individual structures in the skin:

- Capillaroscopy (assessment of the dermal microcirculatory bed)
- Ultrasound scanning (*in vivo* monitoring of structural changes in the dermal layer)

Properly selected cosmetic products can reduce skin discomfort and temporarily improve its appearance but may even eliminate dryness. Conversely, improper moisturizing will, at best, fail to help and, at worst, exacerbate the clinical picture (Draelos Z.D., 2018).

3.1. Emollients: types and properties

Emollients are topical agents that return plasticity and softness to the *stratum corneum*. This broad term applies to preparations that differ in composition and mechanism of action but yield a similar clinical result: skin softening. Let's consider them in more detail.

The main functional ingredients of emollients include three categories of substances:

1. Fatty refractory substances that, after being applied to the skin, remain on its surface and form a water-repellent protective layer (mimicking the sebum function)
2. Lipids that, when applied to the skin, penetrate the *stratum corneum* and are incorporated into the intercellular lipid structures (promoting the lipid barrier restoration and strengthening its structures)
3. Hygroscopic substances that bind and retain water on the surface or inside the *stratum corneum* (serving as "moisture traps")

3.1.1. Lack of sebum and occlusion

Water continuously rises from deep within the skin to the surface and evaporates. If its evaporation is slowed by covering the skin with something gas-tight, the water content of the *stratum corneum* will increase quite rapidly. This method of moisturizing is called occlusive moisturizing.

Sebum is a natural occlusive film, but it is not impermeable. Oxygen and carbon dioxide pass freely through the sebum. Water evaporation is inhibited both by smoothing the horny scales and by the glycerin present in the sebum, but it is not entirely blocked.

A cosmetic product applied to the skin can act as a sebum analog, slowing water evaporation. Ingredients that mimic sebum include:

- Mineral oil, petroleum jelly, liquid paraffin, ceresin — all are hydrocarbons, i.e., petroleum products
- Liquid silicones (silicone oils) are hydrophobic high-molecular-weight organosilicon compounds
- Synthetic waxes, fatty alcohols (octadecanol, hexyl decanol, etc.), fatty esters (decyl oleate, isopropyl myristate, etc.)
- Lanolin (from Latin *Lana* — wool, *oleum* — oil) is an animal wax obtained during the purification of wool wax (it is extracted with organic solvents from sheep's wool)
- Animal fats — goose, whale (spermaceti), pig, badger fats

- Squalene and its derivative *squalane* (from Latin *Squalus* — shark) is a natural component of human sebum; production sources for cosmetic use are different (e.g., shark liver, some plants)
- Vegetable oils, e.g., shea (karite) butter, are primarily refractory and solid
- Natural waxes and their esters — beeswax and vegetable waxes (pine wax, cane wax, etc.)

The above substances belong to hydrophobic moisturizers and differ in occlusion strength, which is the highest for petroleum jelly. In dermatology, it is used for transdermal drug delivery in subacute and deep processes. The disadvantage of petroleum jelly is an unpleasant feeling of heaviness and greasiness. If petroleum jelly moisturizes too well, it can slow down the repair of the epidermal barrier. The cells will not receive the signal in time that the barrier needs "mending."

Primarily occlusive (i.e., preventing water evaporation), moisturizing creams quickly eliminate dry skin symptoms and reduce inflammation and itching caused by different skin diseases. Still, they do not act on the cause of dry skin. If the skin's barrier function cannot be restored (e.g., in atopic dermatitis due to genetic defects), occlusive creams must be used permanently. If there is a chance of recovery, they should be used only at the initial stage and later replaced by products that restore and strengthen the lipid barrier.

3.1.2. Restoration and strengthening of the lipid barrier

For this purpose, lipids that are part of the lipid barrier are included in the formulation of emollients. Once applied to the skin, they quickly penetrate and are incorporated into the intercellular lipid layers, restoring their structure and function. Some part of lipids applied to the skin pass through the *stratum corneum* and reach living keratinocytes, which capture them and further use them to build their lipids or synthesize molecules that serve as regulators of local immunity reactions (Elias P.M., 2022).

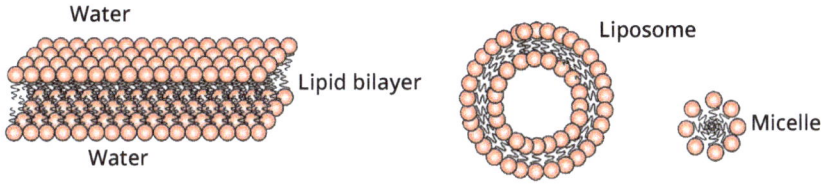

Figure I-3-1. Lipid structures: biological membranes, liposomes, and micelles

Physiologic lipids

Especially effective are lipid mixtures composed of physiological lipids — ceramides (Mutanu Jungersted J. et al., 2010; Choi S.M., Lee B.M., 2015), cholesterol, and free fatty acids. These lipids are physiologic because they constitute the natural lipid barrier of the human *stratum corneum*. It has been experimentally established that an equimolar (i.e., in equal parts) mixture of "fatty acids" has the best restorative properties. It is no coincidence that lipids are among the most popular cosmetic ingredients. They can be included in formulations as individual molecules and structural entities. The latter include, for example, liposomes and micelles (**Fig. I-3-1**). In addition to the traditional role assigned to lipids, such structures act as carriers or containers for other bioactive components, stabilizing them and facilitating their penetration through the *stratum corneum*.

In cosmetics, so-called lamellar emulsions based on phosphatidylcholine (syn.: lecithin) are becoming increasingly popular. Using this technology, tiny lipid droplets are stabilized not by conventional emulsifiers but by a network of bilayers like those that form the lipid barrier (**Fig. I-3-2**). These cosmetics are thus frequently advertised as "preparations structurally conforming to the skin." They have excellent moisturizing and regenerating properties because they resemble the lipid barrier not only in composition but also in structure, which is especially important in the case of dry skin.

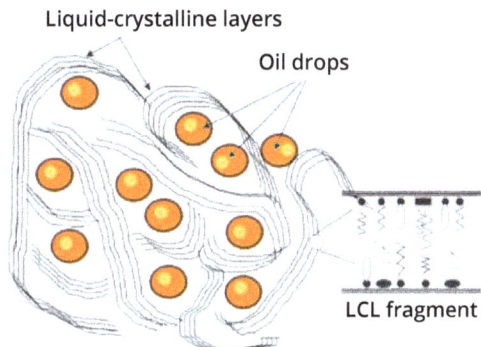

Figure I-3-2. Lamellar emulsion

Natural oils

Natural oils are mixtures of lipids, so their restorative efficacy and preferential mechanism of action depend on their lipid composition.

- **Oils containing essential fatty acids** (linoleic and γ-linolenic acid) promote accelerated synthesis of lipid barrier components, delivering the necessary lipid precursors directly to cells: borage (starflower), evening primrose, and blackcurrant seed oils.
- **Oils rich in sterols** act on living epidermal cells and have anti-inflammatory properties: rosehip, tamanu, soybean, and safflower oils.
- **Oils enriched with saturated and monounsaturated fatty acids** have more pronounced occlusive properties and contribute to the restoration of barrier functions, creating a temporary coating that mimics the action of sebum: shea, tallow, macadamia, corn, coconut, cocoa, and cashew oils.

3.1.3. "Moisture traps" — substances that bind water

Using substances that can bind and hold water molecules (hygroscopic compounds) is a great way to moisturize the skin quickly. Two categories of hygroscopic compounds are used in cosmetics, exerting different effects on the skin.

High-molecular-weight humectants with film-forming and surface humidification properties ("wet compress")

Large polymer molecules (above 3,000 Da) cannot penetrate the *stratum corneum*. They are fixed on the skin surface and absorb moisture like a sponge, forming a "wet compress." Some examples are given below:

- Polyglycols: propylene glycol, ethylene glycol
- Polysaccharides: hyaluronic acid, chitosan, polysaccharides of plant and marine origin (chondroitin sulfate, mucopolysaccharides), pectins
- Polynucleic acids (DNA) and their hydrolysates

- Proteins of animal and plant origin and their hydrolysates (in particular, popular cosmetic ingredients such as collagen, elastin, and keratin are included in cosmetics primarily as moisturizing agents)

Although the listed ingredients are present in almost all cosmetic forms, including emulsions (creams), they are primarily found in gels and liquid products (tonics, lotions, serums, and concentrates). Since hygroscopic polymers do not penetrate the *stratum corneum*, the moisturizing effect is superficial and lasts as long as the polymers hold water on the skin.

In hot and dry climates, applying high-molecular-weight moisturizers to skin with a damaged barrier can even increase TEWL. To mitigate this undesirable effect, products designed for dry skin often combine these substances with occlusive components that prevent water evaporation.

Another option is to use a complementary pair, such as toner plus cream. Applying toner first and cream on top will help soften the skin and retain moisture for extended periods. **The second option is preferred in professional cosmetics, as it offers more possibilities for addressing different skin types individually while considering climatic peculiarities.**

Hygroscopic humidifiers and "deep moisturization"

Several substances can form hydrogen bonds with water molecules, absorbing them from the air and the lower epidermis layers. Water transfer to the overlying *stratum corneum* temporarily increases its hydration.

NMF components, a complex of low-molecular-weight hygroscopic substances, belong to this group. Unlike large high-molecular-weight compounds that remain on the skin surface, NMF components applied as a part of cosmetic products penetrate the *stratum corneum* (but not the lower levels) and increase its water retention potential from within (leading to the so-called "deep moisturizing" effect). As a rule, moisturization that is felt in this case is not so pronounced and does not come as quickly as that imparted by "wet compress," but it lasts longer and depends less on the air humidity.

Hygroscopic "deep" moisturizers include the following substances found in topical products:

- Urea
- Amino acids
- Lactic acid and sodium lactate
- Sodium pyroglutamate
- Glycerin
- Sorbitol trioleate
- Glyceret-26
- Methylglucet-20
- Sorbic acid

Attention! Urea may cause irritation and renal dysfunction in infants. While urea products can be used in toddlers, concentrations are much lower than in adults (Wollenberg A. et al., 2018).

3.1.4. Emollient products

Emollient bases can be anhydrous (ointment, oil) or emulsions (cream, milk, lotion). Ointments are more viscous and are more difficult to spread on the skin than emulsion preparations. The viscosity of emulsions is determined by the ratio of aqueous and oil phases in the preparation, as well as by the substances included in the oil phase. Some examples are given in **Table I-3-1**.

Table I-3-1. Emollients: spreadability and applications

	LOW SPREADABILITY	MEDIUM SPREADABILITY	HIGH SPREADABILITY
Products	• Day and night creams • Eye skincare products	• Day creams and oils • Sunscreens	• Body milk • Hand creams • Bath products
Substances of the oil phase (examples)	• Castor oil • Almond oil • Oleyl oleate • Rice bran oil	• Octyldodecanol • Hexyldecanol • Oleyl alcohol • Decyl oleate	• Isopropyl stearate • Isopropyl palmitate • Isopropyl myristate • Hexyl laurate

3.2. Emollients and the skin microbiome

Using emollients not only improves the skin barrier but also affects the activity of the skin microbiome. As demonstrated by Japanese and Filipino researchers, the use of emollients (twice daily for 1–4 months) led to a 50–78% reduction in the frequency of *S. aureus* excretion from the affected skin of infants and adults with atopic dermatitis (AD) (Verallo-Rowell V.M. et al., 2008; Inoue Y. et al., 2013). Darmstadt G.L. et al. (2014) similarly established that using emollients in preterm infants reduced the risk of skin infections. However, what exactly happens to the microbiome under the influence of this group of products, and, most importantly, why was it not investigated in the studies mentioned above. This knowledge gap prompted Glatz M. et al. (2018) to conduct research on infants at familial risk for AD, some of whom (*n* = 11) had emollient applied to the entire body surface (excluding scalp and diaper-covered areas) from three weeks of age for six months. The control group (*n* = 12) comprising children with similar risks was not treated with emollients. Parents of children in both groups were given the same advice about proper bathing techniques and avoiding soap.

Analysis of the skin microbiome composition at baseline and upon the study completion showed that the emollient group had a significantly higher diversity of bacterial taxa than the control group at all sampling sites (cheeks *p* = 0.002; dorsal surface of forearm *p* = 0.009; palmar surface of forearm *p* = 0.005) (**Fig. I-3-3**). High biodiversity is one of the main attributes of a healthy microbiome. Regarding specific microorganisms, the most significant shift on the skin of infants in the emollient group compared to controls was noted in the *Streptococci*, with a substantial increase in *Streptococcus salivarius*. This microorganism inhabits the skin at birth and has anti-inflammatory effects. *S. salivarius* strains have been shown to reduce the production of pro-inflammatory cytokines and chemokines such as interleukins IL-1β, -6, -8, and tumor necrosis factor-alpha (TNF-α) *in vitro* and to shift the inflammatory response in favor of the T helper 1 (Th1) — an antagonist of the Th2 response characteristic of AD.

The scientists also analyzed skin condition parameters in children from both groups. They found that, in addition to decreased

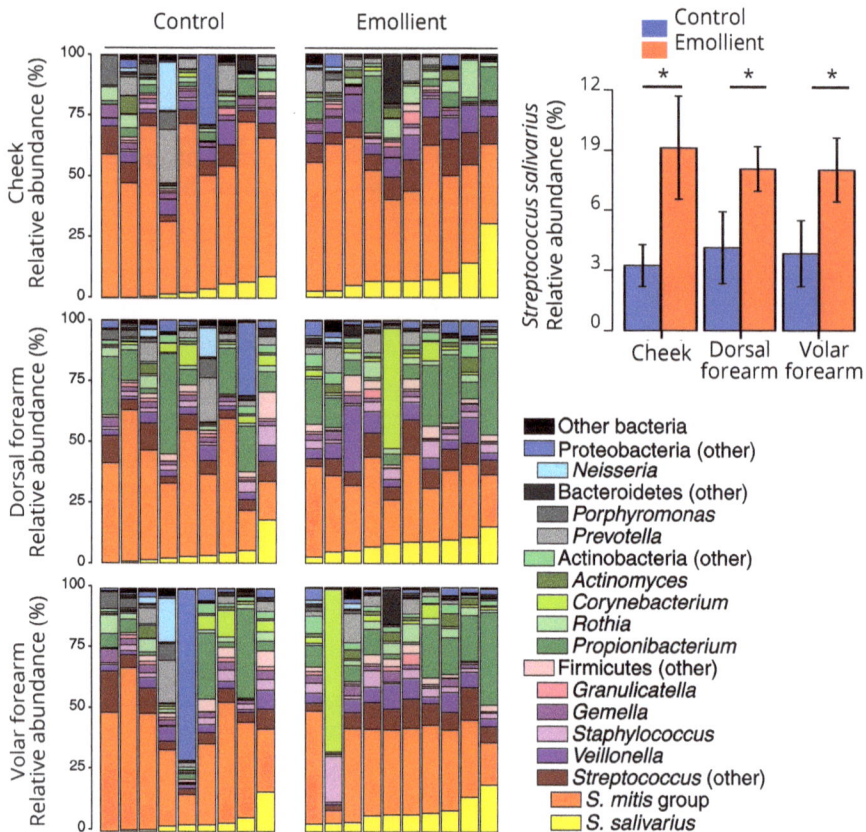

Figure I-3-3. Skin microbiome composition in AD-prone children: with and without emollient use (adapted from Glatz M. et al., 2018)

TEWL and increased hydration, the skin pH in the emollient group was significantly lower than in the control group. There was a moderate correlation between skin pH and the diversity of most microorganisms. However, the authors attributed positive effects in terms of microbiome health to the lowering of pH. They pointed out that some pathogenic organisms, including *S. aureus*, feel much better in conditions of higher pH than in the naturally acidic mantle. But the "good" microflora, particularly *S. salivarius*, prefers acidic pH. Therefore, experts suggest that the change in skin pH is key to the ability of emollients to modify the bacterial communities of atopic skin.

3.3. Climate control

Increasing air humidity is one of the most effective ways to combat dry skin. Prolonged exposure to dry air can deteriorate the *stratum corneum*'s barrier properties, giving rise to dry skin symptoms (Engebretsen K.A. et al., 2018). Air humidity can be increased by using humidifier devices, covering the heating radiators with damp cloths, or placing water containers, plants with large leaves, an aquarium, etc., in the room. If room temperature can be regulated, it should be maintained at the lowest setting that is still comfortable. If air dryness is unavoidable, an emulsion-based moisturizer with emollients and NMF components should be applied to the still-damp skin after each washing or bathing.

The rule "dry air — dry skin" does not always hold. People who have lived in dry climates for extended periods often develop a more effective water-retaining skin barrier compared to those in humid regions, and they do not typically experience dry skin. Generally, skin dryness arises when the skin cannot adapt to a dry environment due to certain congenital traits, significant fluctuations in humidity (such as increased dryness in heated indoor spaces while the outdoor humidity is high), or improper choice of skincare products.

3.4. Moisturizing of pathological skin

Chronic inflammatory diseases such as atopic dermatitis and psoriasis are accompanied by dry skin. Using emollients and moisturizers in these cases reduces discomfort and even dampens the inflammatory response. However, moisturizers and emollients have only recently been recognized as essential in treating psoriasis and AD (van Zuuren E.J. et al., 2017). A complete epidermal barrier cannot be formed in many skin diseases, so the skin does not retain water well while remaining highly permeable to allergenic and toxic substances. Systematic application of products that normalize moisture evaporation from the skin and create a temporary barrier allows the skin to function normally even if the barrier is weak (Schwartz J., Friedman A.J., 2016; Nasrollahi S.A. et al., 2018). The peculiarities of skin moisturizing in atopic dermatitis and psoriasis will be discussed further in Parts II and III.

Chapter 4
Differential diagnosis of dry skin. Algorithm for moisturizer selection

As shown before, quite different pathological mechanisms may be behind a similar clinical picture, so it can be challenging to determine the cause of dryness by eye. Here, instrumental analysis methods that provide objective information about the state of specific skin structures will be of invaluable help (Choi J.Y. et al., 2021).

Armed with diagnostic devices, it is not difficult to measure skin parameters, but it is essential to interpret the results correctly and devise treatment plans based on them. Yet, it is the interpretation that is a stumbling block for many, as it requires extensive knowledge of diverse conditions to conduct a differential diagnosis. Once the diagnosis has been made, we can identify the "weak link" that led to the development of dry skin, allowing us to choose the most optimal strategy for moisturizing the affected skin. For this purpose, at least three parameters should be evaluated (**Fig. I-4-1**):

1. **Hydration (H)** — indicates the water level in the *stratum corneum*
2. **Transepidermal water loss (TEWL)** index — reflects the lipid barrier condition and the extent of its damage
3. **Sebum level (S)** — helps determine sebum activity and the amount of natural emollient on the skin surface

The hydration assessment should confirm that the skin is dry (H↓) and that measures must be taken to moisturize it. Comparing the other two parameters will help us determine which of the skin's water-holding mechanisms is most affected.

Let's look at a few standard situations a skincare practitioner will most likely encounter.

Diagnostic criteria	H↓			
	TEWL↑ / S↔	TEWL↑ / S↑	TEWL↑ / S↓	TEWL↔ / S↔
Causes of dryness	Lipid barrier disruption: • Changes in lipid composition • Partial removal or destruction	Changes in the lipid composition of the lipid barrier as a result of excess sebum	Lack of sebum	NMF deficiency
Skin moisturizing strategy	1. Lipid barrier correction 2. "Wet compress" 3. Occlusion (in damaged barrier)	1. Normalization of sebum production 2. Lipid barrier correction 3. "Wet compress"	1. NMF-containig products 2. "Wet compress" 3. Sebum-like products (occlusion)	NMF-containing products

Figure I-4-1. Algorithm for moisturizer selection based on corneometry, tewametry, and sebumetry: H — *stratum corneum* hydration; S — sebum content; TEWL — transepidermal water loss; ↑ — above normal; ↓ — below normal; ↔ — within normal limits

4.1. Disruption of the *stratum corneum*

If the amount of sebum is within normal limits (S↔) and the TEWL index is elevated (TEWL↑), the epidermal barrier is disrupted. This can occur because of:

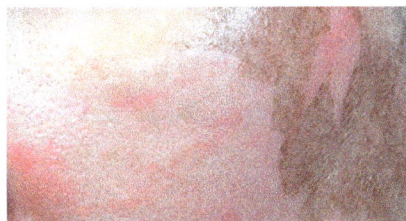

H↓, S↔, TEWL↑

- Trauma, including that caused by aeshetic treatments such as dermabrasion, peels, fractional procedures, and surgery
- Skin disease: psoriasis, atopic dermatitis, ichthyosis
- Changes in the lipid composition of intercellular lipid layers of *stratum corneum*: metabolic disorders due to disease or poor nutrition, long-term use of cosmetic oils with lipids uncharacteristic for the *stratum corneum*, UV radiation (Bak H. et al., 2011)

In case of mechanical damage, preparations with more pronounced occlusive properties (petroleum jelly, lanolin, mineral oil) must be chosen. These products will provide emergency assistance by creating a water-impermeable shield on the skin surface. Due to their application, the skin will maintain the water level necessary for living cells, which generally only survive in an aqueous environment.

Increased TEWL is also observed when the lipid composition of the *stratum corneum* is altered. One of the most common causes of such a condition is a deficiency of essential fatty acids. If the skin's integrity seems intact, but the TEWL is still increased, preparations with essential fatty acids, ceramides, and cholesterol are safe to recommend.

It is possible to change the composition of the lipid barrier by using vegetable oils over a long period. Despite the presence of lipids valuable for the skin, none of the natural oils is a mixture of physiological lipids in the right proportion. Consequently, after application to the skin, the oil penetrates the intercellular spaces and embeds itself in the lipid layers, changing their composition. Consequences depend on the dose:

- If external (exogenous) lipids are scarce, they penetrate the *stratum corneum*, enter the living cells, and are incorporated into fat metabolism.
- Further, the lipids naturally comprising the lipid layers (endogenous lipids) can be synthesized, and the lipid barrier can be assembled.
- If exogenous lipids are too abundant, however, they can significantly alter the composition and properties of lipid layers when incorporated into them. This will disrupt the barrier's lipid lamellar structure and prevent it from adequately regulating water flow.

This analysis leads to a practical conclusion: plant oils, as a source of lipids, should be applied in small quantities to "nourish" the skin occasionally to avoid drying it out after prolonged use. Indeed, ample evidence shows that people who use cosmetic oils for daily care often have dry skin.

In the damaged *stratum corneum*, gel and emulsion preparations with high-molecular-weight compounds (polysaccharides, proteins) acting on the "moisturizing compress" principle can be helpful. They improve subjective sensations and relieve the feeling of tightness. The order of application of moisturizing preparations is of great importance.

Care should be taken when using "wet compress" products, as water evaporates quickly, and gel-forming structural polymers remain on the skin's surface and begin to tighten it. Hence, the "wet compress" product should be covered with an occlusive preparation to prevent the water from evaporating quickly. The exception to this rule is very greasy skin — in this case, the gel "wet compress" is mixed with sebum and does not lose water so quickly.

The order of moisturizer application in case of *stratum corneum* damage:
1. Physiologic lipids
2. "Wet compress" on the emulsion-gel basis (if necessary)
3. Occlusive preparation

4.2. Excessive sebum production

Oily skin often develops dryness, as evidenced by decreased hydration and increased greasiness (oily seborrhea, acne, seborrheic dermatitis). Such skin usually has an elevated TEWL index (TEWL↑), which signals increased lipid barrier permeability due to changes in lipid composition. This may occur be-

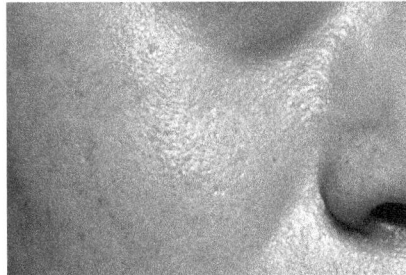

H↓, S↑, TEWL↑

cause the diffusive flow of sebum components through the *stratum corneum*'s intercellular spaces is increased, resulting in a significantly altered lipid profile of the upper layers of the *stratum corneum* (Kircik L.H., 2014).

In this case, preparations for regulating sebum production should be prescribed, such as moisturizing gels "unburdened" by the oil phase and cosmetic vegetable oils containing unsaturated fatty acids. Although water from the "wet compress" will quickly evaporate, this is not a cause for concern because the excess sebum covering the *stratum corneum* will take over the role of the occlusive agent.

The order of moisturizer application in case of dry skin with increased sebum production:
1. Physiologic lipids
2. "Wet compress" on emulsion-gel basis (if necessary)

4.3. Low-sebum skin

Dry skin also develops when sebaceous gland activity is reduced (S↓). This condition is most prevalent in children and older people. Due to sebum deficiency, horny scales are not sufficiently smoothed and literally "become ridged." As a result, the total area of direct contact between the intercellular

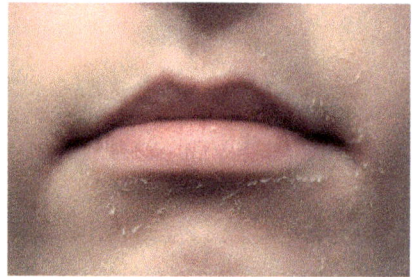

H↓, S↓, TEWL↑

spaces (i.e., the area from which water evaporates) and the air increases. Consequently, water loss through the *stratum corneum* may also increase (TEWL↑).

In this case, dermatologically soft occlusive preparations based on petroleum jelly and mineral oil will effectively correct dry skin. These preparations should contain as few components as possible to avoid adverse skin reactions.

Plant extracts (e.g., chamomile, St. John's wort), bisabolol, and azulene are acceptable components to include in the formulation of anti-inflammatory skincare products.

The order of moisturizer application in case of dry skin:
1. Products with emulsion-based natural moisturizing factor components
2. "Wet compress" on emulsion-gel basis (if necessary)
3. Occlusive preparations that mimic sebum

4.4. Deficiency of natural moisturizing factor

If TEWL and oiliness are within the normal limits (TEWL↔, S↔), but the *stratum corneum* hydration level is nevertheless reduced, the cause may be a deficiency of NMF components. This combination is often observed in atopic dermatitis and other skin diseases associated with keratinization disorders. NMF deficiency can also develop in children before

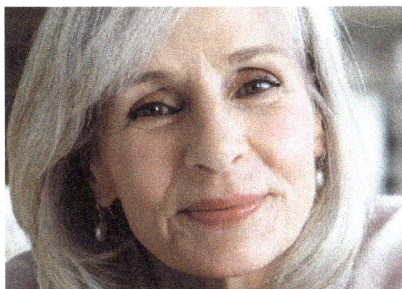

H↓, S↔, TEWL↔

puberty because their epidermis renewal rate is relatively high, so NMF does not have time to accumulate in the right amount in the *stratum corneum*. In older people, NMF decline is due to slower keratinization. Both older adults and children will thus benefit from topical therapy based on preparations that replenish NMF.

NMF components (free amino acids, urea, lactic acid, sodium pyroglutamate) applied to the skin penetrate the surface layers of the *stratum corneum* and partially compensate for the existing deficit (Friedman A.J. et al., 2016). Moisturization provided by NMF molecules is less intensive, but it is longer-lasting compared to the action of film-forming high-molecular-weight polymers. Small molecules easily penetrate and accumulate in the *stratum corneum*, and water bound within it does not evaporate so quickly. Thus, a cumulative effect is observed with regular use of products containing NMF components.

Preparations with NMF are usually based on emulsions containing emollients that soften the skin. Therefore, only one such product will usually suffice for moisturizing.

Applying phytosphingosine is another promising way to increase the NMF level in the *stratum corneum*, as it has been shown to stimulate filaggrin biosynthesis and its subsequent breakdown with the release of NMF components (Choi H.K. et al., 2017).

The order of moisturizer application in case of dry skin with NMF deficiency:
1. "Wet compress" on gel or emulsion-gel basis (if necessary)
2. Cream with NMF (light oil-in-water emulsion)

4.5. General recommendations for skin with increased TEWL

Special attention should be paid to emulsifiers in the prescribed preparation. Even the "mildest" and "dermatologically safe" emulsifiers can penetrate the intercellular spaces, embed in lipid layers, and change their physical and chemical characteristics, which, as a rule, leads to increased *stratum corneum* permeability (James-Smith M.A. et al., 2011).

Skin with the disturbed barrier (due to disease, constant exposure to aggressive substances, UV, and many other reasons) is susceptible to the action of emulsifiers.

Emulsifiers are present in almost every cream (oil-in-water and water-in-oil emulsions). Therefore, if TEWL is high and dryness is very severe, traditional emulsion-based creams should be avoided, and lamellar emulsions or anhydrous occlusive ointments should be prescribed.

Chapter 5
Nutritional features and nutraceutical supplements for dry skin

From a physiological point of view, nutrition involves the ingestion, digestion, assimilation, and metabolism of substances necessary for sustaining life. All body organs and tissues depend on nutrient supply. No organ — even the digestive ones — functions autonomously, and skin is no exception. Nutrients enter the skin through the bloodstream, not from outside, so topical products cannot fully meet its needs. In addition to cosmetic products that replenish fatty acids, NMF, and antioxidants, nutritional changes can help improve skin health.

5.1. Nutrients and dietary intake

Modern recommendations for adjusting dietary intake for people with dry skin are based on numerous studies and clinical observations, some of which are discussed below.

5.1.1. Substances that strengthen the skin barrier

Polyunsaturated fatty acids

As the epidermal lipid constituents, polyunsaturated fatty acids are key in maintaining the skin's barrier function. Omega-3 and omega-6 acids strengthen the *stratum corneum*, promote moisture retention, and prevent transepidermal water loss.

Omega-3, including α-linolenic, eicosapentaenoic, and docosahexaenoic acids, has anti-inflammatory properties, improves skin hydration, and promotes skin repair. Faber C. et al. (2020) demonstrated that omega-3 (eicosapentaenoic acid) at 2 g per day reduced pro-inflammatory cytokine levels in the skin, thus lessening the manifestations of dryness and irritation.

Omega-6, represented by linoleic and γ-linolenic acids, participates in ceramide metabolism — the most essential component of the lipid barrier. Boelsma E. et al. (2003) showed that linoleic acid, an omega-6 constituent, promotes the synthesis of ceramides as the key components of epidermal lipids. Participants who received omega-6 supplements showed improvements in skin elasticity and hydration. However, the authors emphasized the importance of moderate omega-6 intake to avoid competition with omega-3 for enzyme systems.

The importance of maintaining the **correct omega-3/omega-6 ratio**, which should be in the 1:4–1:5 range, has long been recognized (Simopoulos A.P., 2002). Yet, modern diets elevate this ratio to 1:15 or more, contributing to increased inflammation, negatively affecting the skin, and aggravating its dryness and sensitivity. For example, in a study by Kim J. et al. (2018), women who maintained a 1:5 omega-3/omega-6 balance showed improved epidermal structure and increased ability to retain moisture. Those with a predominance of omega-6 (1:15 or higher) suffered from increased skin dryness and inflammation.

Thus, the balance of omega-3 and omega-6 fatty acids plays a key role in maintaining skin health, including hydration, barrier function, and protection against inflammation. For dry skin, increasing the proportion of omega-3 while reducing omega-6 intake is recommended. This can be achieved by consuming oily fish, as well as flaxseed and linseed oil, while minimizing the consumption of foods high in vegetable oils (rich in omega-6).

Antioxidants

Antioxidants are essential dietary components for maintaining healthy skin. Free radicals produced by UV light, pollution, and stress damage cell membranes, compromising the skin's barrier function. Antioxidants such as vitamins E and C, carotenoids, and flavonoids neutralize free radicals, preventing oxidative stress.

Vitamin E protects cell membranes and the lipid barrier from oxidation. According to Schagen S.K. et al. (2012), vitamin E supplementation

(200 mg per day) for eight weeks reduced oxidative stress markers by 30% and skin reactivity in participants with dryness symptoms.

Vitamin C is a water-soluble antioxidant and is also involved in collagen synthesis. In a study by Pullar J.M. et al. (2017) involving 60 participants, vitamin C supplementation (500 mg daily for three months) improved skin hydration and texture. A decrease in wrinkle severity was also observed.

Draelos Z.D. (2020) further established that consuming 500 mg of vitamin C and 200 mg of vitamin E daily for six months improved skin health, reduced redness, and improved texture in people with dry and sensitive skin.

Carotenoids, especially beta-carotene, enhance UV protection by helping to keep the skin moisturized. Based on their analysis of a sample of 50 people, Boelsma E. et al. (2003) noted that a diet high in beta-carotene (15 mg per day) increased skin photoprotection by 40%. Increased *stratum corneum* hydration and decreased inflammation were also observed.

Flavonoids strengthen capillaries, improving microcirculation and maintaining the skin's water balance. An experiment performed by Watson R.R. et al. (2014) showed that daily consumption of grape seed extract containing 150 mg of flavonoids over 12 weeks reduced TEWL by 25%, indicating that the skin's barrier properties were strengthened.

Minerals

Many studies show the importance of minerals in improving dry skin and emphasize the benefits of including them in the diet. Three substances are particularly valuable here — calcium, zinc, and selenium.

Calcium regulates keratinocyte differentiation, restoring the skin barrier function (Lee S.E., Lee S.H., 2018). More than 25 years ago, Green H. (1999) showed that calcium plays a key role in maintaining the epidermal barrier. An experiment involving 60 adults with low dietary calcium levels indicated that increasing calcium intake to the recommended levels (1000 mg per day) for 12 weeks improved skin texture and reduced TEWL by 18%.

Zinc is involved in healing and regulates sebaceous glands, preventing excessive dryness. A study by Rinnerthaler M. et al. (2015) on the effects of zinc confirmed that a daily intake of 15 mg helps accelerate skin regeneration and improve hydration. Participants noted a reduction in the sensation of dry skin after as little as four weeks of regular zinc supplementation.

Selenium is an antioxidant that protects the skin from oxidative stress by reducing damage caused by external factors. For example, Zouboulis C.C. and Makrantonaki E. (2022) observed decreased oxidative stress markers and increased skin elasticity in a group that took 55 µg of selenium daily for three months.

5.1.2. Substances that impair skin barrier

Eliminating several substances from the diet helps to improve skin hydration and repair.

Trans fats found in margarine, fried foods, and fast food disrupt the skin's lipid barrier, making it more susceptible to external damage (Barcelos R.C. et al., 2015).

Regular consumption of sugar-rich food contributes to skin aging and dryness symptoms; in contrast, reducing sugar intake improves skin turgor and hydration, which becomes noticeable after eight weeks (Zouboulis C.C., Makrantonaki E., 2022). Thus, a diet conducive to glycation products accumulation is another factor that negatively affects skin hydration. Glycation is a non-enzymatic process in which sugars modify proteins and lipids. Accumulation of glycated keratin in the epidermis is accompanied by decreased *stratum corneum* hydration and contributes to skin dryness (Sakai S. et al., 2005). The cause may be excessive binding of glucose to connective tissue fibers of the dermis, resulting in a decrease in the skin's elasticity and moisture retention capacity (Yokota M., Tokudome Y., 2016). Such an adverse effect of glycation on skin hydration has been observed in people with diabetes mellitus, which is explained by the increased level of glycation end products associated with this disease (de Macedo G.M. et al., 2016). For instance, in their study involving 49 patients with diabetes with fasting plasma glucose levels above 110 mg/dl, Sakai S. et al. (2005) found that the degree of skin hydration was lower compared to patients with glucose levels below 110 mg/dl without apparent changes in TEWL.

Excessive alcohol consumption negatively affects the skin — it causes dehydration, thins the skin barrier, and increases inflammation, elevating the skin cancer risk (Yen H. et al., 2017).

5.2. Nutraceuticals based on hyaluronic acid and collagen

In addition to a balanced diet, people with dry skin should take nutraceuticals containing hyaluronic acid and collagen, which form the skin's intercellular matrix.

Hyaluronic acid is known for its ability to retain moisture. Filling the intercellular space in all skin layers is vital for maintaining the skin's water balance. Hyaluronic acid supplements are increasingly recommended to improve dry skin symptoms. A randomized controlled trial by Yamada Y. et al. (2022) demonstrated that taking 120 mg of hyaluronic acid daily for eight weeks increased the skin hydration levels by 24% compared to a placebo. Study participants also noted a reduction in the feeling of skin tightness.

Special attention should be paid to **collagen hydrolysates**, as many studies have demonstrated that oral intake helps restore skin hydration and reduce fine lines and wrinkles (Dewi D.A.R. et al., 2023). For example, a randomized study conducted by Proksch E. et al. (2021) confirmed that collagen hydrolysate not only improves the quality of the dermal matrix but also helps to strengthen the skin barrier and increase the skin's resistance to external factors, which is especially relevant for people with chronic dry skin. de Miranda R.B. et al.'s (2021) meta-analysis of 19 studies with 1,125 participants aged 20 to 70 provides a complete picture of the systemic administration of collagen peptides on skin hydration. The reported results confirm the positive impact of systemic administration of hydrolyzed collagen on skin hydration and signs of photoaging.

5.3. Probiotics

A healthy microbiome is one of the guarantors of maintaining the integrity of the epidermal barrier and ensuring optimal skin hydration.

The most straightforward and accessible tools for building a healthy microbiome are probiotics.

Probiotics are live microorganisms that benefit health when administered in adequate amounts. Probiotics have been reported to improve skin health and prevent acne, as well as allergic and atopic dermatitis (Dolan K.E. et al., 2017).

In a randomized study by Lee D.E. et al. (2015) involving 110 patients aged 41–59 years with dry skin and significant signs of photoaging, the participants were divided into the experimental (n = 81) and the placebo (n = 29) group. Patients in the experimental group received *Lactobacillus plantarum* HY7714 at a daily dose of 10^{10} colony-forming units (CFUs) for 12 weeks. Skin hydration on the back of the hand and face was measured at 4-week intervals. Compared to the baseline, TEWL scores after 4, 8, and 12 weeks were significantly reduced in both groups. However, after 12 weeks, only participants in the experimental group showed a significant increase in skin hydration.

Similarly, Mori N. et al. (2016) studied the skin hydration dynamics in 101 healthy young women for the first four weeks, after which the participants were divided into two groups. The first (experimental) group included 81 participants who drank a probiotic preparation containing *Bifidobacterium breve Yakult* (YIT 12272), *Lactococcus lactis* (YIT 2027), *Streptococcus thermophilus* (YIT 2021), polydextrose, and galacto-oligosaccharides daily for four weeks. The remaining 20 participants (the control group) did not consume the probiotic drink. After four weeks of probiotic supplementation, the *stratum corneum* hydration level increased from a baseline of 23.2 to 25.1 in the experimental group. In the control group, no significant changes in skin hydration were recorded.

More recently, Kim H.S. et al. (2020) showed that probiotic supplementation with *Bifidobacterium lactis* for eight weeks improved skin hydration and promoted skin microbiome restoration in winter climate conditions.

5.4. General recommendations for food rationing

To reduce dry skin symptoms, it is recommended to avoid foods containing saturated animal fats and trans fats (hydrogenated fats that are poorly absorbed by the body). This means limiting the consumption of red meat, fatty poultry, and "junk food" (chips, hamburgers, etc.).

To improve the condition of dry skin, increasing the consumption of foods rich in polyunsaturated fatty acids is recommended, maintaining a balance between omega-3 and omega-6. Optimizing the diet by introducing antioxidants such as vitamins E and C, carotenoids, and flavonoids helps reduce inflammation and restore the skin's barrier function. Including foods containing calcium, zinc, and selenium helps speed up regeneration and protects the skin from oxidative stress. Eating oily fish such as salmon, cod, and mackerel is beneficial. Fish is a source of polyunsaturated fatty acids, essential for the immune system and for building the lipid barrier. In addition to fish, vegetable oils — corn, rapeseed, olive, and linseed — are recommended, as they are rich in valuable fatty acids. A salad of shredded cabbage and carrots dressed with oil, as well as fruits (citrus fruits, apples, etc.) and berries (sea buckthorn, blueberries, grapes, etc.), are excellent sources of antioxidant vitamins.

Although all nutrients are best obtained from food, supplements containing essential fatty acids, antioxidants, and minerals in known dosages can ensure the body receives the necessary amounts of these substances.

Nutritional supplements with probiotics, hyaluronic acid, and collagen hydrolysate are effective nutraceutical tools for improving dry skin symptoms. They can be included in a dry skin correction program along with other measures, such as a balanced diet and topical products, for better results.

Finally, drinking enough water and maintaining proper nutrition is vital for hydrating skin.

The peculiarities of nutrition for patients with atopic dermatitis and psoriasis are described in Parts II and III.

Part II

Atopic dermatitis

Chapter 1
Etiology and pathogenesis

Atopic dermatitis (AD) is a chronic inflammatory skin disease affecting individuals with a hereditary predisposition. According to different sources, its prevalence ranges from 2.1% to 4.9% in adults and from 2.7% to 20.1% in children (Zuberbier T. et al., 2023). The disease manifests within the first six months of life in 45% of patients and by the age of five in 85%. Only half of children with AD experience persistent remission in adulthood (Czarnowicki T. et al., 2017).

The most critical components of AD etiopathogenesis are:

- Genetic predisposition
- Imbalance in the skin microbiome
- Aggressive environmental factors (UV, cold temperatures, low humidity, strong wind, etc.)
- Structural and immunologic abnormalities of the epidermal barrier leading to increased TEWL

Increased TEWL associated with greater *stratum corneum* permeability is a characteristic feature of affected and unaffected skin of AD patients (Çetinarslan T. et al., 2023). Enhanced TEWL rate correlates with the disease severity. Dry skin, one of the hallmarks of AD, occurs due to increased water loss and leads to pruritus, significantly impairing the quality of life of atopic patients.

There are two key links in the AD pathogenesis:

1. Immune dysregulation
2. Impaired barrier function of the skin

The question of which one is the primary contributor is still open.

According to the traditional ideas about AD pathogenesis, the first place is occupied by abnormal T cells, which enter the dermis through the bloodstream and provoke an inflammatory reaction. Inflammation disrupts the epidermis's homeostasis, resulting in the *stratum corneum* not forming correctly and ceasing to cope with the barrier function. In other words, damage to the *stratum corneum* stems from inflammation. According to this "inside-out" scenario, if inflammation is extinguished, the homeostasis of the overlying layers is restored. Therefore, the therapy primarily relies on anti-inflammatory agents, corticosteroids, and immunosuppressive drugs (e.g., calcineurin inhibitors).

In contrast, the "outside-in" scenario suggests that abnormal *stratum corneum* is the first link in the pathogenetic chain. Foreign agents enter the skin through a weak barrier, and the immune system responds to inflammation. If this is the case, it is worth strengthening the *stratum corneum* with the help of a corneotherapeutic approach, as the symptomatology will be reduced, and long-term remission can be attained in some cases.

Both scenarios share common mechanisms that lead to chronic inflammation. Below, we will discuss each mechanism as a potential target for therapeutic intervention.

1.1. The "outside-in" scenario, or primary disruption of the epidermal barrier

The "outside-in" scenario implies that barrier disruptions facilitate the penetration of various allergens, irritants, and microorganisms into the skin of atopic patients, triggering a cascade of inflammatory responses with a corresponding clinical picture. This assumption is supported by extensive evidence (Czarnowicki T. et al., 2017).

The skin barrier structures localized within the *stratum corneum* (corneocytes, lipid barrier) and on its surface (hydrolipid mantle) are impaired in AD patients.

Atopic patients exhibit several characteristic genetically determined changes in the epidermal barrier that underlie the clinical symptoms of AD, such as skin dryness and inflammation (**Fig. II-1-1**).

1.1.1. Mutations in genes encoding filaggrin

Filaggrin is a major epidermal structural protein synthesized by keratinocytes in the upper layers of the epidermis. The breakdown products

CORNEOCYTES ("BRICKS")	INTERCELLULAR LIPIDS ("MORTAR")	CORNEODESMOSOMES ("BRIDGES")
Filaggrin- and loricrin-encoding genes' mutations ↓NMF (PCA, urocaninic acid, free amino acids) Changes in corneocyte shape	Changes in the activity of enzymes responsible for the assembly of lamellar lipid structures Changes in lipid composition: ↓ Ceramides ↓ Sphingosine (anti-microbial substabce) ↑ Cholesterol sulfate ↓ Cholesterol ↓ Free fatty acids	Increased activity of enzymes destroying corneodesmosomes
H↓	TEWL↑	Scaling

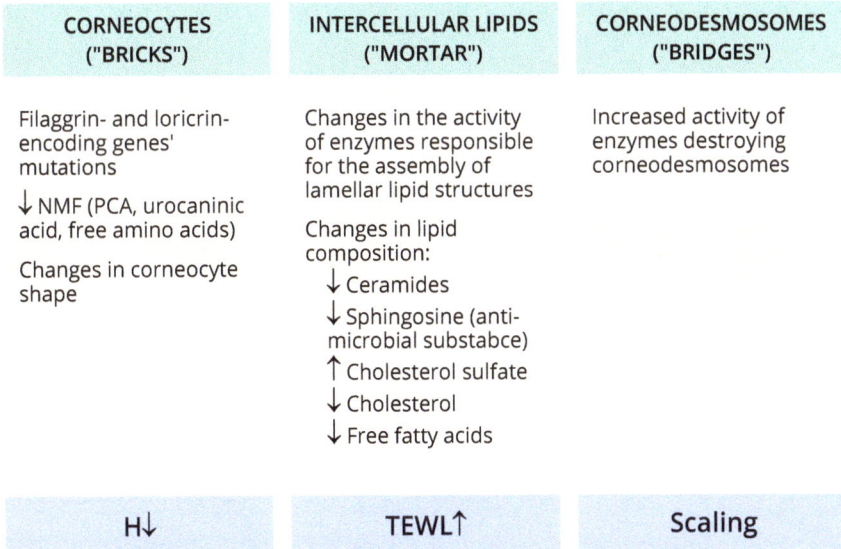

Figure II-1-1. Genetically determined changes in the lipid barrier of the *stratum corneum* in atopic dermatitis

of filaggrin maintain the acid–base balance and provide optimal skin hydration and antimicrobial protection (Kim Y., Lim K.M., 2021).

Mutations in the gene encoding filaggrin (*FLG*), disrupting the filaggrin structure, are a significant risk factor for AD. They occur in 30–50% of light-skinned atopic patients (Patrick G.J. et al., 2021). Genetic abnormalities of the filaggrin structure are accompanied by decreased NMF content, increased TEWL index, and impaired skin elasticity and strength (**Fig. II-1-2**). In addition, they are associated with increased allergic sensitization and may lead to earlier disease onset, more severe course, and higher prevalence of bronchial asthma, food allergies, and microbial infection.

Laboratory studies on mouse models of AD indicate that not only does the structure of keratinocytes change against the background of filaggrin deficiency, but the production of lipid precursors comprising the lipid barrier of the *stratum corneum* also decreases (Elias M.S. et al., 2017), which negatively affects its barrier function.

In the skin of atopic patients, there is a decrease in the production of epidermal antimicrobial peptides and consequent alteration of the skin

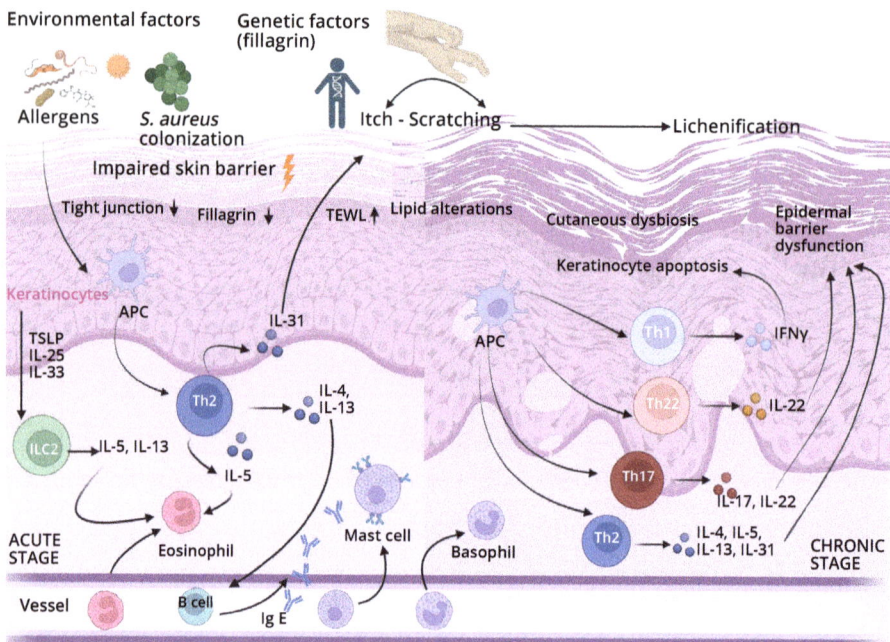

Figure II-1-2. Immunopathogenesis of atopic dermatitis. Acute and chronic stages of AD (adapted from Çetinarslan T. et al., 2023)

Abbreviations: APC — antigen-presenting cell; IFN — interferon; IgE — immunoglobulin E; IL — interleukin; ILC2 — type 2 innate immune lymphoid cell; TEWL — transepidermal water loss; Th — T helper cell; TSLC — thymic stromal lymphopoietin cell

microbiome (Langan S.M. et al., 2020); in particular, increased skin colonization by *S. aureus* has been identified (Clausen M.L. et al., 2017).

In addition, *FLG* mutation is associated with an increased risk of early disease onset, high serum immunoglobulin E (IgE) levels, persistence of AD into adulthood, and other manifestations of atopy (Zaniboni M.C. et al., 2016).

Yet, such clinical signs are found in only 10–40% of atopic patients, and up to 40% of people with an *FLG* mutation are clinically healthy. Everything depends on the type of mutation — to date, about 40 variants of *FLG* mutations have been identified in European and Asian populations.

Most children with manifestations of AD eventually enter a persistent remission. This fact indicates that, in addition to *FLG*, other genes may be involved in the AD manifestation (Czarnowicki T. et al., 2017).

1.1.2. Defects in corneodesmosomes and tight junctions

Congenital corneodesmosome defects lead to skin barrier disruptions. Desquamation occurs after the destruction of the corneodesmosomes' extracellular part. Alterations in various corneodesmosome components (e.g., desmoglein-1) contribute to AD pathogenesis.

Atopic patients also have a congenital deficiency of transmembrane tight junction proteins, which is especially pronounced in the presence of mutations in the filaggrin gene. The level of claudin-1 decreases, and the more pronounced the claudin-1 deficiency, the more significant the increase in skin barrier permeability (Czarnowicki T. et al., 2017).

1.1.3. Changes in the lipid barrier and hydrolipid mantle composition

Intercellular lipid layers act as a barrier against pathogen penetration and maintain the *stratum corneum* integrity (Elias P.M., 2005). The optimal ratio of *stratum corneum* lipids is one condition that ensures the integrity of the epidermal barrier. Changes in the quantitative and qualitative composition of the lipid barrier characterize AD. Dysfunction of the epidermal barrier can be caused by mutations in genes responsible for enzymes that metabolize lipids, and such mutations can lead to increased protease activity or decreased protease inhibitor activity.

In AD, ceramide levels typically decrease (Levin J. et al., 2013). The immune/inflammatory response influences ceramide metabolism in AD. Inflammatory cytokines (IL-4, -13, and -31) reduce the expression of key enzymes required for ceramide formation (Danso M.O. et al., 2017). For instance, van Smeden J. and Bouwstra J.A. (2016) demonstrated a characteristic decrease in total ceramide levels and changes in ceramide structure characteristic of AD:
- An increase in short-chain ceramide levels and a decrease in long-chain ceramide levels
- An increase in short-chain free fatty acid levels and a decrease in long-chain free fatty acid levels
- A decrease in fatty acids with hydroxyl group levels

These characteristic changes in the lipid barrier are a feature of atopic skin and are not limited to the rash area (Toncic R.J. et al., 2020). Due to unfavorable changes in the epidermal lipid qualitative and quantitative composition due to AD, the TEWL increases, and skin hydration decreases.

Atopic skin is also characterized by sebum deficiency, contributing to dryness and increased irritability. These conditions are essential in AD pathogenesis (**Table II-1-1**).

Table II-1-1. Genetically determined changes in sebum composition in patients with atopic dermatitis

LIPID SPECIES	HEALTHY SKIN	ATOPIC SKIN	CHANGES IN AD
Squalene	12.8 ± 0.6	10.8 ± 1.1*	↓
Choelsterol	1.2 ± 0.2	2.4 ± 0.4*	↑
Cholesterol esters	1.3 ± 0.2	2.4 ± 0.6*	↑
Wax esters	25.6 ± 3.2	21.7 ± 1.8*	↓
Triglycerides	36.1 ± 8.4	32.6 ± 10.6	downward trend
FFAs	21.6 ± 8.8	28.8 ± 11.4	upward trend
Diglycerides	1.4 ± 0.2	1.3 ± 0.2	no changes
TOTAL	195.4 ± 20.6	172.6 ± 17.4*	↓

* Statistically significant result compared to healthy skin, $p < 0.05$

1.1.4. Changes in skin surface pH

To preserve the integrity of the skin barrier, lipid metabolism, keratinocyte differentiation, and antimicrobial defense, it is necessary to maintain a slightly acidic pH of 4–6 on the skin surface. Evidence from several studies indicates that the skin pH of atopic patients is usually neutral or even slightly alkaline, which is somewhat related to the deficiency of filaggrin breakdown products (Czarnowicki T. et al., 2017). Increased pH affects the ratio of microbial flora components on the skin surface, facilitating their multiplication. Under conditions characterized by increased pH, serine proteases of the *stratum corneum* are activated, leading to accelerated corneodesmosome destruction and increased desquamation (Barton M., Sidbury R., 2015).

These changes cause the epidermal barrier of atopic skin to lose its functional integrity, making restoration and maintenance mandatory. **Table II-1-2** summarizes the main components of skin barrier dysfunction in AD.

Table II-1-2. Disruption of the epidermal barrier in AD

FUNCTION	STRUCTURE	CHANGES IN AD
Water regulation	• Lipid barrier • NMF	• Disturbances of lamellar strata structure and TEWL enhancement • Reduced NMF content associated with a genetic defect in filaggrin synthesis
Mechanical barrier	• Corneocytes • Corneodesmosomes	• Abnormal corneodesmosome breakdown • Changes in the corneocyte shape
Chemical and antimicrobial barrier	• Lipid barrier • Hydrolipid mantle	• Changes in lipid composition • Increase in pH
Renewal of the *stratum corneum*	Enzymes of the *stratum corneum* (proteases, glycosidases)	• Increased activity of proteolytic enzymes against the background of increased pH • Acceleration of desquamation and thinning of the *stratum corneum*

1.2. The "inside-out" scenario, or immune dysregulation

In this mechanism of AD manifestation, the genetically mediated feature of the immune response to allergens is of primary importance.

The leading triggering role in AD is played by:

- Aeroallergens (house dust mites, mold, animal hair, pollen, etc.)
- Live pathogens (*Staphylococci*, dermatophyte fungi)
- Contact chemical allergens
- Food allergens

Food allergens are the primary triggers in infancy; in adult patients, polyallergy predominates, with food allergens losing importance.

According to the hygiene hypothesis of AD pathogenesis, disease development is associated with reduced microbial exposure in early childhood due to the emphasis on high levels of household hygiene in recent decades (cleanliness of the living areas, frequently changed clothes, bedding, and towels, daily washing, limiting contact with animals, etc.). The consequence of this stringent hygiene regimen is a lack of early immune system stimulation, which "teaches" it to resist environmental allergens and microbes.

AD was previously considered a Th2-mediated inflammatory disease because most patients have increased serum IgE levels and high quantities of circulating eosinophils. However, recent evidence suggests a T-cell biphasic response (Tokura Y., Hayano S., 2022).

Th2 cell activity predominates at all stages of AD. Direct exposure of the skin of an AD patient to a causative allergen activates antigen-presenting cells of the epidermis — Langerhans cells. These cells migrate to the lymph nodes, activating Th2 lymphocytes, which begin to secrete pro-inflammatory cytokines and chemokines (IL-4, -5, -10, -13, -31). This group of mediators is involved in allergic reactions, switching B cells to IgE production, disruption of terminal differentiation of keratinocytes (through the inhibition of filaggrin, loricrin, and involucrin), and suppression of antimicrobial peptides, which leads to increased skin permeability to exogenous antigens and pathogens.

Th1 activation is observed in later stages, leading to increased IFN-γ levels and eventually keratinocyte apoptosis (Chovatiya R., Silverberg J.I., 2019). It has been reported that the inflammation in rash foci in the chronic stage of AD is due to a complex interaction between T helper cells (Th1/Th2/Th17/Th22) and hyperproliferative keratinocytes with altered terminal differentiation (Renert-Yuval Y. et al., 2021).

Moreover, the immune response in AD is characterized by eosinophilia, increased spontaneous histamine release from basophils, and chronic activation of macrophages with heightened secretory activity.

It should be noted that defects in the innate immune response result in a lack of microbial growth restriction and contribute to susceptibility to colonization and infection by *S. aureus*.

1.3. The role of human microbiome in atopic dermatitis

Progress in understanding the microbiome and its role in human health is considered one of the most significant achievements of modern biology and medicine. In 2007, the U.S. National Institutes of Health initiated a large-scale *Human Microbiome Project*, bringing together scientists from around the globe. The results of these international studies have led to profound changes in views on human biology and the development of many diseases, including dermatologic diseases.

According to the accumulated data, microorganisms living on the surface of our skin participate in its defense and contribute to maintaining homeostasis. **Changes in the microbial landscape can be both a cause and a consequence of skin pathology.**

1.3.1. Gut microbiome

Atopic patients exhibit abnormalities in the species composition and diversity of the skin and gut microbiome (De Pessemier B. et al., 2021). However, whether these changes result from gut/dermal barrier disruption and inflammation or their cause is still unclear.

At the same time, an interrelationship between commensal microorganisms and the immune system has been established. Changes in the microbiome's species composition are believed to affect the formation of innate and acquired immunity at an early age.

Colonization of the child's gut with bacteria begins at birth; the species composition of the microbiome rapidly expands until the infant is 2–3 years old, after which the flora becomes like the adult flora (Arrieta M.C. et al., 2014).

The mode of delivery has a pronounced effect on the development of the gut microbiome in youth (Fujimura K.E. et al., 2010). During birth through the natural birth canal, the infant encounters the maternal vaginal microflora consisting of commensal organisms often found in the lower gastrointestinal tract (Tannock G.W. et al., 1990). *Bifidobacterium* and *Bacteroides* strains characteristic of the microbiome of these children contribute to the maintenance of health and suppression of inflammatory responses. In children born by cesarean section, *Streptococci*, *Staphylococci*, and *Clostridium difficile* strains predominate in the microbiome (Penders J. et al., 2006).

Infant feeding methods — artificial and breastfeeding — strongly influence the gut microbiome in early life. In artificially fed infants, *Escherichia coli* (*E. coli*) and *Clostridium* (e.g., *C. difficile*) are common in the gut flora, whereas in breastfed infants, *Bifidobacterium* strains dominate (Klaassens E.S. et al., 2009). The introduction of solid food causes a dynamic shift in the intestinal microflora from *Bifidobacterium*-dominant to *Bacteroides*- and *Clostridium*-dominant composition (Valles Y. et al., 2014).

Colonizing the gut with bacteria at an early age (during the first three years of life) has a pronounced effect on the human immune system, affecting health later in life. Proper immune system development is highly dependent on gut bacteria, as evidenced by the loss of immune function in laboratory-sterile mice lacking a microbiome. Previous animal and human studies have shown that gut flora and their metabolites (e.g., short-chain fatty acids, SCFAs) are actively involved in the proliferation and differentiation of both B and T cells.

As we approach the age of 70, the function of digestion and absorption of nutrients in the gut changes, which affects the composition of the gut microbiome. Decreased immune system activity in the elderly leads to weakened defense against pathogens, contributing to changes in the overall microbiome. Since *Bifidobacterium* strains modulate immune system activity and metabolic processes, their decreased abundance may lead to nutrient deficiencies and a pro-inflammatory background in older people. The commensal flora requires favorable conditions, depending on the body's general state. Changes in the microenvironment are accompanied by alterations in the composition and diversity of the microbiome, which can lead to disease (Aggarwal N. et al., 2023).

Several studies have been devoted to the microbiome of atopic patients. According to one such investigation, the number and proportion of *Bifidobacterium* in atopic patients was significantly lower than in healthy individuals (Watanabe S. et al., 2003). In addition, the number and proportion of *Bifidobacterium* in the gut microbiome differed according to disease severity, with lower values found in patients with severe AD. In contrast, *S. aureus* was more prevalent in AD patients than in healthy individuals.

Numerous studies have confirmed that gut dysbiosis precedes the onset of AD (Lee S.Y. et al., 2018). It has also been observed that children with AD lack bacterial diversity, in addition to low amounts of *Bifidobacterium* and *Bacteroides* and high levels of *Enterobacteriaceae* and *Clostridium* (Nylund L. et al., 2015).

Significant dysbiosis of *F. prausnitzii* species was found in fecal samples from atopic patients (Song H. et al., 2016). A concomitant decrease in SCFAs, which help maintain the integrity of the epithelial barrier and exert anti-inflammatory effects, was also observed. Increased intestinal mucosal permeability in atopic patients promotes skin inflammation by allowing toxins, poorly digested food, and microbes to enter the systemic bloodstream (**Fig. II-1-3**). A strong Th2 response is initiated when they reach the skin, causing significant tissue damage (Kim J.E., Kim H.S., 2019).

The gut microbiome also forms the skin flora. SCFAs (i.e., propionate, acetate, butyrate) are the end products of dietary fiber fermentation in the gut. They are known to play an essential role in shaping the composition of the skin microbiome, which is closely linked to cutaneous immune defense mechanisms (Salem I. et al., 2018). *Cutibacterium* produces SCFAs such as acetate and propionic acid in the gut. Propionic acid and its esterified derivatives inhibit the growth of methicillin-resistant *S. aureus* strain USA300 under *in vitro* conditions (Schwarz A. et al., 2017). Moreover, cutaneous commensals such as *S. epidermidis* and *C. acnes* tolerate broader changes in SCFA levels than other strains. Together, these findings suggest a close interaction between the gut and skin.

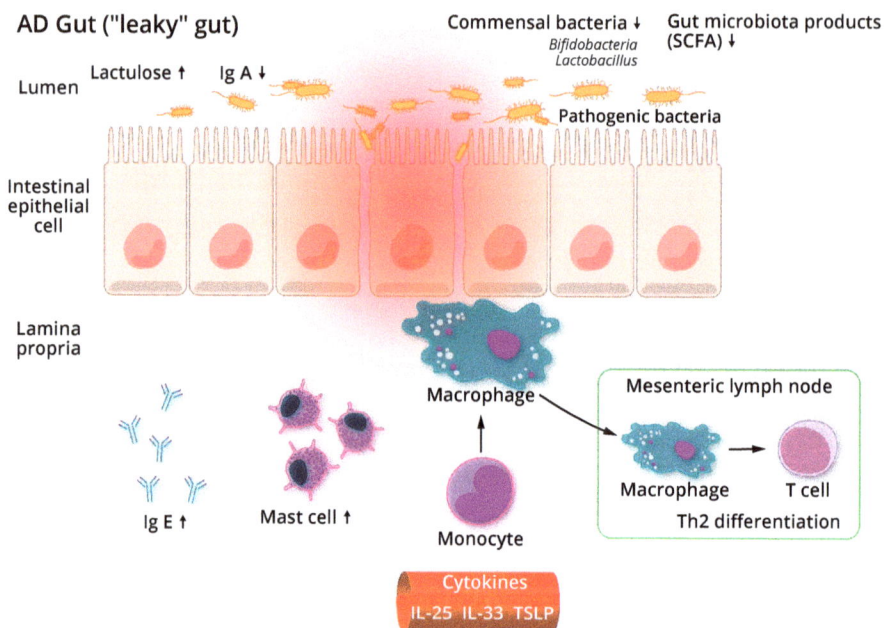

Figure II-1-3. Disruption of the intestinal mucosal barrier in AD (adapted from Kim J.E. et al., 2019)

Patients with AD are characterized by dysbacteriosis and decreased intestinal short-chain fatty acid levels. In response to pro-inflammatory cytokines, monocytes migrate and differentiate into macrophages. Antigen penetration through the mucosa from the intestinal lumen converts T cells to Th2 cells in the draining lymph nodes. Immunoglobulin E (IgE) and mast cells are also more prevalent in the intrinsic lamina of the mucosa

1.3.2. Skin microbiome

The skin of atopic patients exhibits several specific changes in the microbiome's species composition compared to healthy individuals' skin (**Fig. II-1-4**) (Hrestak D. et al., 2022). However, whether these changes are due to epidermal barrier dysfunction and immune dysregulation is unclear.

Although the species composition of the skin microbiome is highly dependent on the anatomical region, elevated numbers of different *Staphylococci* strains, especially *S. aureus*, have been observed in AD (Moniaga C.S. et al., 2022). It has been reported that *S. aureus* is present on the skin in 30–100% of atopic patients and only 20% of healthy individuals (Paller A.S. et al., 2019). According to the meta-analysis

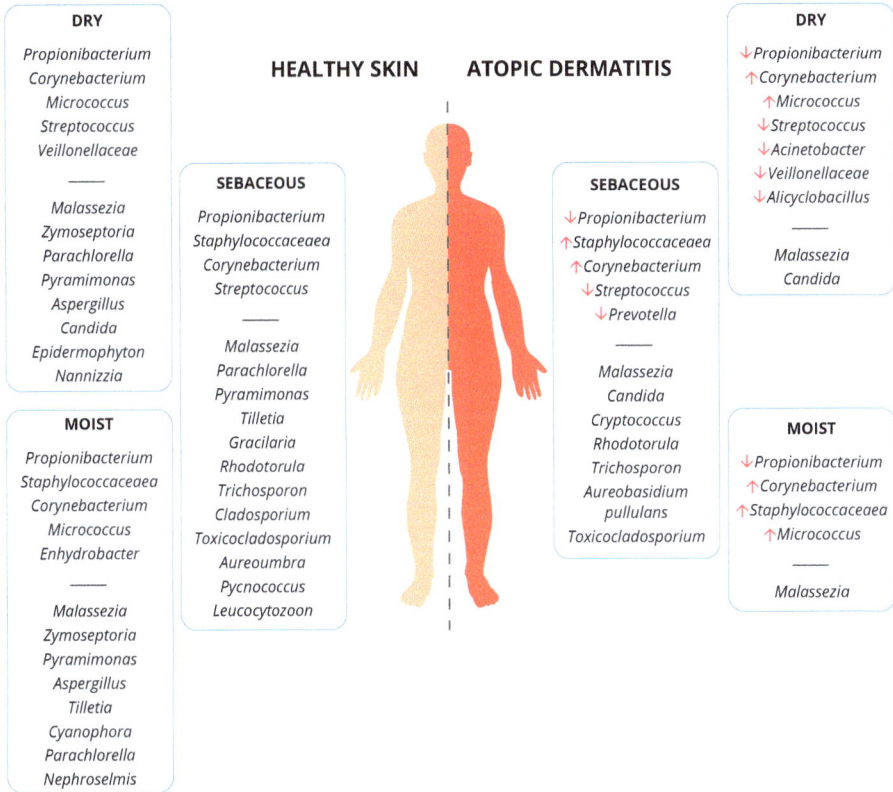

Figure II-1-4. Comparison of the skin microbiome of a patient with atopic dermatitis and a healthy person (adapted from Hrestak D. et al., 2022)

conducted by Totte J.E. et al. (2016), the proportion of *S. aureus* in the skin microbiome varies even in the same AD patient. It ranges from 39% on skin without rash elements to 70% on skin with rash elements. In the presence of genetic mutations affecting filaggrin, often found in AD, breakdown products of this protein, such as urocanic acid and pyroglutamic acid, are usually produced in smaller quantities, resulting in an increase in pH that promotes *S. aureus* proliferation. Increased pH can also enhance the virulence of *S. aureus* by modulating the expression of several proteins involved in adhesion and evasion of the immune response (e.g., agglutination factor, fibronectin-binding protein), allowing *S. aureus* to colonize the skin of atopic patients even more actively (Miajlovic H. et al., 2010).

AD Skin

Commensal ↓ Filaggrin ↓

Corynebacterium
Cutibacterium
CoNS

AMP ↓

Biofilm CoNS *S. aureus* CoNS

<SC Lipid>
CER[EOH]C66 ↓
CER[EOH]C68 ↓
FFA 16:1 ↓
FFA 18:1 ↓

TEWL ↑ pH ↑

Epidermis
— Corneum
— Granular
— Spinous
— Basal

LC

Kallikreins ↑

S. aureus toxin

IL-4
IL-5
IL-13

Cytokines
TNF-α
IL-1
TSLP

Induce Th2 cell differentiation

IgE ↑ Eosinophils ↑ CCL17 ↑

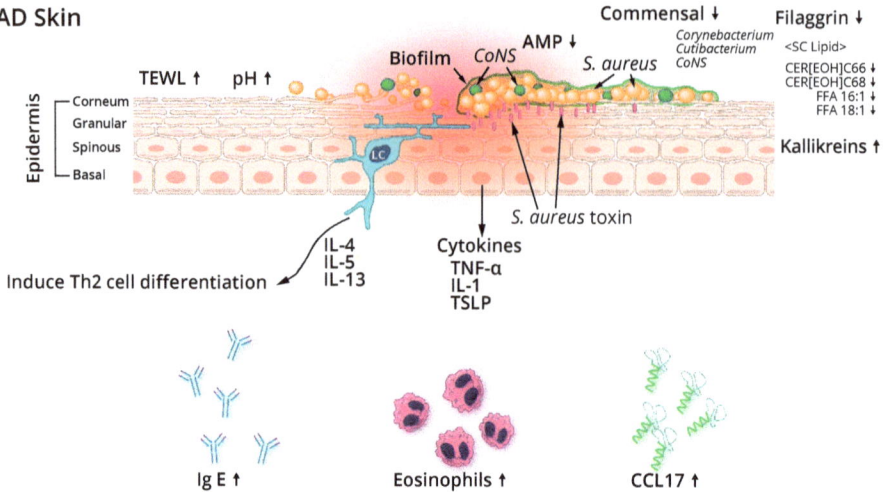

Figure II-1-5. Disruption of the epidermal barrier in atopic skin

The density of *S. aureus* infestation correlates with the severity of the disease regardless of localization. Thus, *S. aureus* is present in greater quantities in chronic rashes than in regions with acute rash and visually unchanged skin. The skin flora shows low microbial diversity during AD exacerbation regardless of age. In atopic patients, skin sites with inflammatory rash elements are characterized by a decrease in *Cutibacterium*, *Streptococci*, *Acinetobacter*, *Corynebacterium*, and *Prevotella* (**Fig. II-1-5**) along with an increase in *Staphylococci* (Kong H.H. et al., 2012; Kim J.E., Kim H.S., 2019). In addition to *S. aureus*, in AD, other *Staphylococci* species (*S. epidermidis* and *S. haemolyticus*) are common at sites with rash elements (Gonzalez M.E. et al., 2016).

S. aureus strains isolated from atopic lesions differ from those isolated from unaffected skin. Some *S. aureus* proteins can attach to the *stratum corneum* molecules. For instance, Fleury O.M. et al. (2017) reported that, in severe AD, strains with clonal complex 1 (CC1), which provides tight attachment to the *stratum corneum*, are more frequently isolated from the skin surface. In contrast, strains with clonal complex 30 (CC30), characterized by a lower ability to adhere, are more frequently isolated in mild AD manifestations. Adhesion ensures the formation of biofilm — a bacterial community consisting of cells attached to the surface or each other and embedded in a matrix of extracellular polymers.

Biofilm formation plays a vital role in the chronic persistence of *S. aureus* on the skin in AD and prevents the elimination of these pathogens by antibiotics. *S. aureus* biofilm grows rapidly on the epidermis, causing oxygen deprivation and impairing the skin's protective barrier function (Lone A.G. et al., 2015).

1.3.3. *S. aureus* in the AD pathogenesis

The mechanisms contributing to skin colonization by *S. aureus* involve complex interactions among several factors (Koh L.F. et al., 2022):

- Damage to the skin barrier
- Reduction of lipid content in the skin
- Skin surface pH alteration in the alkaline direction
- Defective innate immune responses due to the decreased production of endogenous antimicrobial peptides

Two major endogenous antimicrobial peptides in human skin exist: β-defensins and cathelicidins. These peptides are produced by keratinocytes and act against bacteria, viruses, and fungi. According to one proposed mechanism, the antimicrobial action of defensins is due to damage to the pathogen's cell membrane, disrupting intracellular functions. After gaining access to the skin, *S. aureus* colonies grow uncontrollably without antimicrobial peptides.

Over 70% of isolated *S. aureus* can produce exotoxins, including staphylococcal enterotoxins A, B, and C (SEA, SEB, SEC) and toxic shock syndrome toxin-1 (TSST-1). These exotoxins act as superantigens, penetrate the epidermal barrier, and aggravate inflammation. Many studies emphasize the relationship between *S. aureus* colonization and AD severity (Nowicka D., Grywalska E., 2018).

Microbial contamination with *S. aureus* has a toxic effect on keratinocytes, stimulates lymphocyte interferon secretion, and consequently leads to chronic disease. The bacteria themselves and their metabolites trigger activation of T lymphocytes, macrophages, and antigen-presenting cells, leading to increased IgE and IgG production. High IgE levels are a characteristic symptom of an immune response to an allergen.

Another well-known factor in AD pathogenesis is impaired epidermal lipid metabolism. This condition leads to changes in the percentage of free fatty acids, ceramides, and cholesterol in the *stratum corneum* as well as affects the skin microbiome. Baurecht H. et al. (2018) investigated the relationship between microbiome diversity and epidermal lipid composition. Their analyses revealed that high levels of unsaturated long-chain FAs were associated with increased *Cutibacterium* and *Corynebacterium* quantities. In contrast, high levels of saturated short-chain FAs were associated with a decrease in the abundance of these genera. These authors also found an association between high ceramide CER-(AS) levels and increased *S. aureus* abundance. Levels of some ceramides such as CER(AH)C38-C52 and CER(AP)C40 — especially long-chain ceramides CER(EOH)C66-C70 and CER(EOS)C70, some triglycerides, and unsaturated FAs — were significantly lower in atopic patients with positive *S. aureus* colonization status than those without such a condition (Li S. et al., 2017). These studies revealed an interesting relationship between epidermal lipid composition and microbiome structure in AD.

Many mechanisms contribute to the colonization of the epidermal surface by *S. aureus*, and at the same time, many processes induced by these microorganisms aggravate the course of the disease. Thus, *S. aureus* colonization is both a cause and a consequence of the disease.

1.4. Psychoneuroimmunology of atopic dermatitis

Stress and neuroendocrine factors may be involved in the onset, recurrence, or worsening of several dermatologic diseases. These effects appear to be mediated by neurohormones, neuropeptides, and neurotransmitters that modulate interactions between the skin, nervous, immune, and endocrine systems.

A clear correlation between stress and allergic skin conditions has not yet been found, and it cannot be stated that stress can trigger an allergic reaction under all circumstances. However, some people with a genetic predisposition may develop such conditions.

Stress can induce AD by disrupting the skin barrier function and promoting a switch in immune response to a Th2-lymphocyte response (Arndt J. et al., 2008). These changes may underlie the disease pathogenesis. In addition, chronic stress can reduce the activity of natural killer (NK) cells, leading to increased susceptibility to infections and exacerbation of skin diseases (Moynihan J.A., 2003).

Another hypothesized pathogenetic mechanism in AD is increased reactivity of the sympathetic–adrenal system, leading to an imbalance between the adrenergic and cholinergic systems and a clinically pronounced paradoxical vasoconstriction in response to mechanical skin irritation (Buske-Kirschbaum A. et al., 2006).

In chronic stress, the initial adaptation mechanisms are directed toward coping with the stressor. They stimulate the secretion of various neuropeptides and neurohormones that play an essential role in the onset and development of the disease. For example, the secretion of catecholamines and cortisol, the primary stress hormones, significantly affects the immune system. They inhibit IL-12 production by antigen-presenting cells that stimulate Th1 cell response (Elenkov I.J., Chrousos G.P., 1999). Besides, corticosteroids directly stimulate the Th2 response, increasing IL-4, -10, and -13 production (Mizawa M. et al., 2013).

Thus, **chronic stress may induce an imbalance in Th1/Th2 responses, favoring a Th2-mediated reaction. Impaired neuroimmune homeostatic mechanisms may also promote the emergence of an allergic inflammatory response.**

Stress also modulates cutaneous nerve fibers. In addition, atopic patients experience significant changes in the plasma and tissue levels of neuropeptides such as vasoactive intestinal peptide (VIP), nerve growth factor (NGF), substance P (SP), and neuropeptide Y (NPY).

Another neuropeptide that may be involved in AD pathogenesis is calcitonin gene-related polypeptide (CGRP). SP, CGRP, and VIP cause vasodilation and increased vascular permeability at higher levels. The action of SP on monocytes and macrophages increases TNFα and IL-12 production, while CGRP stimulates Langerhans cell function to initiate Th2 immune responses (Abdelhadi S. et al., 2024). In addition, SP and corticotropin-releasing hormone released at the peripheral level during inflammatory flares induce mast cell degranulation, thereby exacerbating symptoms.

Mast cells may be another link between stress and AD exacerbation, not only via stressor-induced mast cell degranulation but also by increasing their number in the skin (Căruntu C. et al., 2014). Plasma levels of histamine and its concentration in the skin of atopic patients are also increased.

The skin microbiome is another target for stress. Stress is known to exacerbate pruritus via the skin–brain axis. As a result, the microbiome is increasingly considered a major regulator of interactions along this axis, especially during stress. The communication pathways between the microbiome and the brain are gradually being elucidated (Kim H.S., Yosipovitch G., 2020). Stress acts through the central nervous system (CNS) and alters the microbiome by releasing neurochemicals. Components of the stress response, such as glucocorticoids, can inhibit AMP release in the epidermis and contribute to impaired skin barrier properties and increased susceptibility to pathogens. Members of the skin microbiome, especially coagulase-negative staphylococci, are sensitive to catecholamines. Catecholamines also increase bacteria's ability to adhere and their virulence, creating favorable conditions for biofilm formation by *Pseudomonas aeruginosa* and *Escherichia coli*, which increases the virulence of methicillin-resistant *S. aureus*. Norepinephrine, epinephrine, dopamine, and structurally related inotropes (dobutamine and isoprenaline) increase *Staphylococci* growth by five or more times. Thus, the effect of stress on the skin microbiome can be twofold: weakening the host defense against infectious agents and creating an ideal microenvironment for pathogens (Radek K.A., 2010).

Based on this evidence, it can be surmised that numerous neuropharmacological agents, such as neuropeptides (NPY, VIP, SP, CGRP), neurotransmitters (acetylcholine, norepinephrine, serotonin, histamine, glutamic acid, γ-aminobutyric acid), and hormones (adrenaline and glucocorticoids), are involved in modulating neuronal receptors that enhance inflammation.

Chapter 2
Clinical presentation and diagnosis

2.1. Clinical picture

The clinical manifestations of AD depend on age.

Infancy

The infancy (the period spanning from 2–3 months to 2 years of age) is characterized by bright hyperemia, symmetrically located exudative rashes, wetting, and crusts, predominantly localized on the face, buttocks, and extensor sides of the shins and forearms. By 1.5–2 years of age, rashes move to the typical sites for this disease — the neck, elbow bends, hamstring fossa, wrists, ankle joints, and the back of the feet (Katoh N. et al., 2020). Triggers at this age are mainly foods, most commonly milk and cereals.

Childhood

In childhood (from 2–3 years to puberty), there are changes in the rash localization and appearance, whereby follicular and lichenoid papules, infiltrative, erythematous-squamous foci, excoriation, and dyschromia prevail. Rashes are mainly located on the elbow bends, wrists, the hamstring fossa, and the neck. The skin becomes dry, pale, and mottled, and areas of secondary post-inflammatory pigmentation alternate with hypopigmented regions. Some children develop atopy stigmas — periorbital hyperpigmentation and Dennie–Morgan folds* (**Fig. II-2-1**).

---

* A Dennie–Morgan fold, also known as a Dennie–Morgan line or an infraorbital fold, is a fold or line in the skin below the lower eyelid. It can simply be an ethnic/genetic trait, but it was found in one study to occur in 25% of patients with atopic dermatitis (Wikipedia).

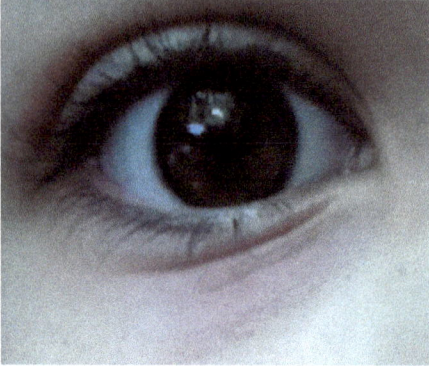

Figure II-2-1. Dennie–Morgan fold below the lower eyelid (adapted from Wikipedia)

Aeroallergens become more critical than food factors. This period is characterized by the seasonality of exacerbations, coinciding with the fall–spring period, and the resolution of rashes in summer, especially in southern resorts. During an exacerbation at any age, lymphadenopathy with involvement of cervical, inguinal, and axillary lymph nodes may be observed.

Adolescence and adulthood

In adolescence and adulthood, infiltration, lichenification, excoriated lichenoid papules, skin fissures, and dyschromia predominate (**Fig. II-2-2** and **II-2-3**). The rashes are predominantly below the knees, on elbow folds, wrists, and hands (**Fig. II-2-4**). The skin is susceptible to

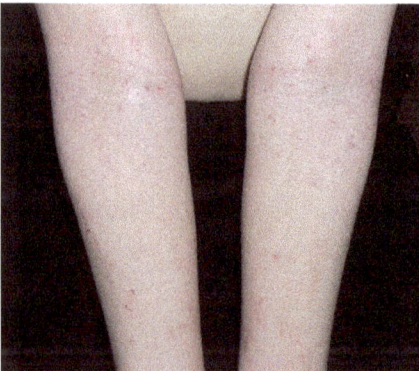

Figure II-2-2. Excoriated papules, lichenification (photo provided by V.I. Albanova)

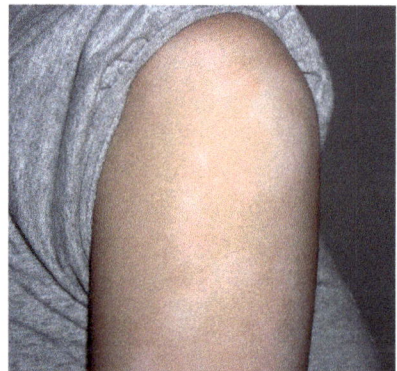

Figure II-2-3. Dyschromia (photo provided by V.I. Albanova)

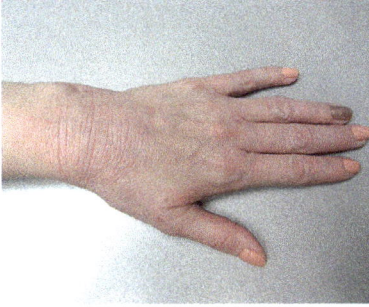

Figure II-2-4. Hand lesions (photo provided by V.I. Albanova)

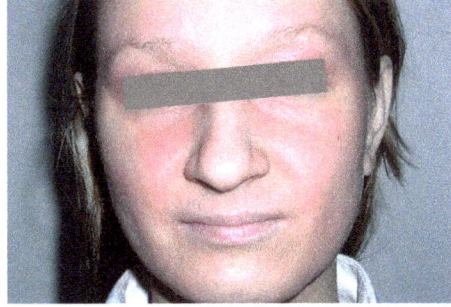

Figure II-2-5. Intolerance to cosmetic cream in a patient with AD (photo provided by V.I. Albanova)

contact irritants, and allergic reactions are frequent. The hands become affected, with clinical manifestations typical of eczema.

In adult patients, skin dryness and lichenification dominate the clinical picture. Atopic patients are also characterized by high sensitivity to cosmetics (**Fig. II-2-5**) and foods. All these symptoms are practically independent of the season.

The peculiarities of adult patients are related to the fact that they are "tired of treatment" and "know better than any doctor what to do." They stop visiting a dermatologist, rarely use systemic drugs, apply topical glucocorticosteroids (GCSs) at any redness (often failing to choose those that are modern and safe), neglect skincare, and fail to adhere to the rules on limiting sun exposure. Long-term use of topical GCSs invariably affects the skin, leading to atrophy, dryness, telangiectasia, acne, redness of exposed areas, and early signs of aging.

Most patients have a mild or moderately severe disease course (limited rashes, rare exacerbations, moderate pruritus). In rare cases of severe AD, rashes are widespread and poorly amenable to therapy; remissions are short-lived, lasting no more than 1–1.5 months.

The most frequent complications of AD include secondary infection with bacteria (especially *S. aureus*), fungi (*Candida*, *Malassezia*), and viruses (*herpes simplex*, papillomas). Bacterial infection often results in folliculitis and impetigo, while furuncles and viral infection (common warts, *molluscum contagiosum*) are less common. Kaposi's herpetic eczema and mycotic infection (pruritus, cheilitis, vulvovaginitis, *Malassezia folliculitis*) are rare.

2.2. Diagnostic criteria and differential diagnosis

2.2.1. Diagnostic criteria

AD is diagnosed based on historical and clinical features, the typical morphology and distribution of skin lesions, and the exclusion of other dermatoses. Hanifin J.M. and Rajka G. (1980) proposed the diagnostic criteria for AD, which have since been expanded (Jeskey J. et al., 2024). According to the current guidelines, diagnosing **AD requires three major and three minor criteria**.

Main features (three or more must be present)
- Pruritus
- Typical clinical picture and localization of rashes
- Chronic recurrent course
- Presence of concomitant atopy (bronchial asthma, allergic rhinitis, conjunctivitis)
- Early age of onset
- Personal or family history of atopy
- Presence of allergen-specific IgE in the medical history, actually or expected (in children aged below 12 months) in the peripheral blood and/or skin

Pruritus is a hallmark of AD, and the diagnosis should be reconsidered in its absence.

Minor (less-specific) features
- Dry skin (xerosis)
- Ichthyosis
- Atopic palms (creasing and dryness of the palms, palmar hyperlinearity)
- Follicular keratosis
- Keratosis pilaris
- Tendency to allergic dermatitis and eczema of hands and feet (in adults)
- Persistent white dermographism

- Frequent pyoderma
- Frequent *herpes simplex* episodes
- Recurrent conjunctivitis
- Atypical vascular changes (facial plethora, perioral pallor, white dermographism, delayed blanching)
- Dark circles under the eyes
- Rarefaction of the lateral portion of the eyebrow
- Infraorbital folds (Dennie–Morgan folds)
- Ocular changes (keratoconus, anterior subcapsular cataracts)
- Cheilitis
- Geographic tongue
- Folding of the anterior surface of the neck
- Retinal pigmentation on the neck (the "dirty neck" symptom)
- White lichen
- Secondary leukoderma
- Nipple eczema
- Susceptibility to cutaneous infections (especially *S. aureus* and *herpes simplex*) and impaired cell-mediated immunity
- Immediate (Type I) skin test response
- Drug allergies
- Urticaria
- Increased itching at night and sweating
- Provoking influence of emotional, nutritional, climatic, infectious, and other factors
- Seasonality in symptom severity

2.2.2. Differential diagnosis

The differential diagnosis should be made for adult patients with the following diseases.

Seborrheic dermatitis

In seborrheic dermatitis, the skin is oily; there are no excoriations of lichenification. Rashes in seborrheic dermatitis are characterized by hyperemia and excessive scaling in zones rich in sebaceous glands — on the face (interbrow area, cheeks, nasolabial folds, behind the ears), scalp, chest, and interscapular area; itching is rare and weak.

Allergic dermatitis

Allergic dermatitis is caused by repeated contact with an allergen to which sensitization has developed. Rashes in the form of erythema, swelling, papules, and vesicles may appear not only at the site of contact with the allergen but also at distant sites. With proper treatment, the rash resolves quickly. It differs from AD due to predominantly exudative rash, lack of typical localization, lichenification, and stigmas of atopy. Allergic dermatitis is often combined with AD.

Contact dermatitis

Contact dermatitis is limited to rashes at the site of irritant exposure (high and low temperatures, sunburn, solutions of alkalis, acids, and other substances). The erythema's brightness, swelling, blisters, and erosions depend on the irritant's toxicity and resolve spontaneously after the exposure ceases.

Scabies

Scabies is a contagious skin disease (acrodermatitis) caused by the *Sarcoptes scabiei* mites. It is transmitted from person to person through prolonged direct skin-to-skin contact. Scabies is characterized by the involvement of the palms and soles in the inflammatory process, the presence of large nodules in the skin folds (cutaneous lymphoplasia), predominantly nighttime itching, no effect on itch from antipruritic agents and topical GCSs, and the presence of similar manifestations of the disease in other family members.

Microbial eczema

Microbial eczema is a clinical type of eczema that is secondary to microbial or fungal skin lesions. It is characterized by adding inflammatory changes characteristic of eczema to the symptoms of the existing background disease. The disease onset is related to the violation of skin integrity (scratches, abrasions, wounds). Due to improper treatment, papules, pustules, wetting, and crusts occur on an erythematous background. Rashes merge into asymmetric plaques typically located on the back of the hands, forearms, shoulders, shins, and thighs, and less often on the trunk.

Psoriasis

Psoriasis is a chronic, non-infectious autoimmune disease affecting mainly the skin. In psoriasis, lesions in the form of plaques with clear boundaries and silver scales on the surface are primarily localized on the scalp, elbows, knees, face, and perineal area; itching is slight or absent. In the initial stage, rashes can exist for a long time as a single focus on the face or scalp. For more information on psoriasis, see Part III.

Autosomal dominant ichthyosis

Autosomal dominant ichthyosis (also known as ichthyosis vulgaris) is a group of inherited skin diseases characterized by keratinization disorders. It can be present alongside AD. Early generalized skin desquamation is observed, which is more pronounced on the lower legs while absent from skin folds. Symptoms include creasing of the palms and soles (indistinguishable from atopic palms) and the absence of inflammatory changes and itching (except in combination with AD). Family history helps with the correct diagnosis.

Mycosis fungoides at the erythematous stage

Mycosis fungoides (also known as Alibert–Bazin syndrome or granuloma fungoides) is the most common form of cutaneous T-cell lymphoma. It usually affects the skin but can eventually spread to internal organs. Symptoms include rashes, tumors, skin lesions, and severe itching. In the erythematous stage, itchy erythematous patches with indistinct scaling appear on the skin, resembling manifestations of AD. Differential diagnosis is essential to analyze the history of the disease (absence of rashes in childhood), the lack of rashes typical for AD, and lichenification.

Chapter 3
Basic skincare

Disruption of the epidermal barrier (perceived as "dry skin") is a core characteristic of AD. Hence, restoration of the skin barrier function is central to AD management, regardless of the disease severity, and is aimed at correcting keratinization abnormalities as well as abnormalities in the lipid composition of the *stratum corneum* and reducing TEWL (Wollenberg A. et al., 2023). In practice, this treatment is often called "skincare," mistakenly believing it is different from or less critical than medical interventions. However, it should be remembered that optimal care for atopic skin can prolong remission and alleviate or even eliminate rashes.

3.1. Skin cleansing

Skin cleansing is an integral part of AD skincare. However, it must be done correctly to prevent disruption of the skin barrier, worsening of disease symptoms, and the formation of microenvironmental conditions favorable to pathogens.

Studies show that prolonged exposure to water can cause damage to the *stratum corneum*, typically accompanied by increased skin permeability and susceptibility to irritants and infections (Herrero-Fernandez M. et al., 2022). Besides, increases in TEWL may also occur due to water evaporation from the skin surface after bathing, exacerbating skin dryness and irritation. In recent years, clinicians have attempted to identify optimal bathing parameters such as duration, frequency, water temperature, and special cleansers to maximize the therapeutic effect.

3.1.1. Frequency, temperature, and duration of bathroom procedures

Most international guidelines recommend a daily bath of 5–10 minutes with warm water, followed by emollient application. On the other hand, there is no consensus on the optimal water temperature. For instance, according to the European and Korean consensus guidelines for treating AD, bath water should be in the 27–30 °C range, while the Japanese guidelines stipulate 36–40 °C (Kim J.E. et al., 2015). The rationale behind these recommendations is that itching occurs at 42 °C and higher skin temperatures, and 36–40 °C is optimal for restoring the skin barrier function (Katoh N. et al., 2020).

The frequency of washing procedures also matters. According to Rakita U. et al. (2023), showering/bathing more than once a day is associated with higher scores on AD clinical severity scales such as o-SCORAD (Scoring Atopic Dermatitis), SCORAD-itch, EASI (Eczema Area and Severity Index), POEM (Patient-Oriented Eczema Measure), and DLQI (Dermatology Life Quality Index). These authors observed AD symptom attenuation (according to the o-SCORAD, EASI, and POEM measures) with regular and even patchy application of moisturizer after shower/bath. The duration of shower/bathing did not affect the clinical manifestations of AD. Thus, showering/bathing daily or less frequently and applying moisturizer immediately after is associated with lower AD severity, whereas shower/bathing duration has no significant effect on AD symptoms.

3.1.2. Special cleansers

There is no consensus on incorporating cleansers into the skincare regimen for atopic patients. On the other hand, most soaps have an alkaline pH. They can worsen the typically higher pH of atopic skin and increase protease activity, leading to epidermal barrier dysfunction. In AD, syndets are preferred for skin cleansing.

Syndets are synthetic detergents with mild surface-active agents (surfactants), physiological pH values, reduced irritation potential, and lack of sensitizing properties. They are capable of maintaining or restoring the cutaneous acid mantle. The surfactant type determines the cleanser's irritation potential. Anionic surfactants, often found in cheap cleansers, have the highest irritation potential. Non-ionic and amphoteric surfactants have a gentler cleansing effect.

Findings yielded by several studies comparing the efficacy of cleansing the skin with special cleansers and plain water indicate that atopic patients may not benefit from cleansers. For example, Inuzuka Y. et al. (2020) noted that washing with water alone was not inferior to washing with soap in maintaining eczema remission in pediatric patients with well-controlled AD. In an earlier study, Noviello M.R. and Italian Pediatric Group (2005) found that cleansing with pure water was comparable to cleansing with syndet or a mild liquid baby cleanser to maintain the acid mantle and reduce sebum on the skin surface. Considering these findings, the American Academy of Dermatology (AAD) consensus guidelines for AD therapy recommend limited use of neutral or acidic pH (5–6), hypoallergenic and fragrance-free soaps or non-soap cleansers (syndets, aqueous solutions) because of their better tolerability (Eichenfield L.F. et al., 2014). In the case of bathing, natural oils can be added to the water in the last two minutes to prevent dehydration of the *stratum corneum*. Adding sodium chloride at concentrations up to 5% to bathing water containing oil is recommended because of its keratolytic and moisturizing effects (Hon K.L. et al., 2016). In adults, magnesium-enriched salt in higher concentrations may be combined with UV irradiation to mimic the effects of balneotherapy.

Although bath additives have gained popularity among patients with inflammatory skin diseases, their clinical benefits remain unclear. It is believed that bath supplements may have therapeutic effects when used in conjunction with mainstream treatments (**Table II-3-1**) (Maarouf M. et al., 2019; Pagliaro M. et al., 2024).

Table II-3-1. Bath additives used in atopic dermatitis (Pagliaro M. et al., 2024)

ADDITIVE	EFFECTS	APPLICATION	INDICATIONS
Sodium hypo-chlorite (whitening baths)	Reduction in the severity of AD manifestations due to antimicrobial activity, ability to modulate the surface microbiome without causing antibiotic resistance, as well as antipruritic and anti-inflammatory effects.	Sodium hypo-chlorite (Na-OCl) should be diluted in bathing water at a 0.005% concentration	The European Consensus Guidelines and the American Academy of Dermatology Guidelines recommend the use of sodium hypochlorite in patients with moderate to severe AD with frequent infectious complications. The Japanese consensus guidelines are more cautious about the use of sodium hypochlorite because of the limited evidence base.
Baby skin cleansers	Removal of impurities and sebum from the skin surface, maintenance/restoration of the skin's acid mantle.	Syndets with neutral or acidic pH, hypoallergenic and fragrance-free products	Recommended for AD in the European, American, and Japanese guidelines.
Bath oils	Formation of a lipid film on the skin normalizes TEWL and reduces NMF loss.	Adding oil to bathing water	The European guidelines recommend adding oils to the water in the last two minutes of bathing; they do not specify which bath oil should be used (mineral, lanolin, vegetable, oatmeal).
Bath salts	Removal of dead cells in the presence of crusts and rough skin. For example, Dead Sea water containing magnesium chloride (MgCl) helps to keep the skin moisturized, has a positive effect on the proliferation and differentiation of the epidermis, and reduces inflammation in AD.	Adding salt to bathing water	Can be used in combination with narrowband ultraviolet B (nbUVB) phototherapy. The use of other salts, such as MgSO and NaCl, in AD requires further study.

Continued on p. 100

ADDITIVE	EFFECTS	APPLICATION	INDICATIONS
Rice starch	Reduction in the severity of erythema, flaking and itching. Presumably, the starch penetrates the upper layers of the skin and fills microcracks, forming a homogeneous layer.	10 g/l, 15 minutes twice a day for four consecutive days	Lack of efficacy studies
Citric acid	Increases skin hydration, suppresses inflammation and colonization of the skin by pathogens (especially *Pseudomonas*).	Adding citric acid to bathing water	Lack of studies
Acetic acid (vinegar)	Reduction of eczema manifestations, antibacterial action	Adding vinegar to bathing water	Lack of efficacy studies
Green tea extract	Reduces itching and severity of AD manifestations	Adding green tea to bathing water	Lack of efficacy studies
Tannin	Anti-inflammatory, antioxidant, antibacterial, antimutagenic, and anticarcinogenic effects	Adding tannin to bathing water	Lack of efficacy studies
Sodium hydrogen carbonate	Antibacterial and anti-pruritic properties	Adding sodium bicarbonate to bathing water	Lack of efficacy studies

3.1.3. General recommendations for skin cleansing in atopic dermatitis

- The bath/shower frequency should not exceed once a day
- The optimal duration of washing procedures is about 5–10 minutes

- Alkaline cleansers containing irritants (anionic surfactants, alcohol, acetone, preservatives, fragrances) should be avoided
- Using detergents with neutral or acidic pH (pH 5–6) is recommended
- When cleansing the face, it is possible to use micellar solution, thermal water, and cleansing milk (oil-in-water emulsion). The milk is applied to the skin with light massaging movements and is rinsed off with water or wiped off with a cotton pad
- Dermabrasion (with sponges, loofahs, scrubs, etc.) must be avoided
- In secondary infection, baths with sodium hypochlorite solution may be helpful
- Adding oils to the water in the last two minutes of bathing is recommended
- Even after a short bath, emollients should be applied to still-wet skin

3.1.4. After-cleansing skincare

Once the skin is exposed to water, its barrier properties are further weakened, and its permeability to external agents increases. However, serious consideration should be given to whether the skin needs more active ingredients in its deeper layers, whether this will increase the likelihood of rapid development of adverse reactions, and whether auxiliary substances will penetrate the skin, causing allergic reactions and other unwanted effects.

It seems more appropriate to apply emollients to the skin immediately after washing and medications 20–30 min later. Individuals with severe AD should use topical GCSs capable of more active penetration, given several reports that prolonged (20 min) bathing followed by application of topical GCSs to wet skin has a more pronounced anti-inflammatory effect in such cases (Gutman A.B. et al., 2005; Hajar T. et al., 2014). To promote more active penetration of topical GCSs, a wet compress is sometimes used (after bathing, topical GCSs are applied to the skin, which is covered by a damp cloth with a dry cloth on top).

3.2. Emollients are the primary topical agents for softening, moisturizing, and protecting atopic skin

Emollients are the mainstay of therapy for any form of AD. However, using pure oil products such as coconut or olive oil instead of emulsions dries the skin and increases TEWL, so they are not recommended.

3.2.1. Emollient composition

According to the consensus opinion of European dermatologists, the ideal emollient contains five key components (Proksch E. et al., 2020):
1. Moisturizers
2. Non-physiological lipids (mineral or vegetable oil)
3. Physiological lipids (ceramides, free fatty acids)
4. Antipruritic/soothing agents
5. Substances that improve epidermal differentiation, as well as dexpanthenol

Physiological lipids (ceramides and free long-chain fatty acids, in particular) are necessary to maintain the adequate composition and organization (orthorhombic packing) of the lipid barrier of the *stratum corneum*. Introducing physiological lipids into the emollient composition increases the proportion of lipids forming orthorhombic (very dense) structures, thus improving the barrier function of dry skin.

Mineral and vegetable oils (i.e., non-physiological lipids), which provide an occlusive effect on the skin surface, are another critical component of emollients for dry atopic skin. They improve the functioning of enzymes involved in NMF metabolism and desquamation, which do not work when the skin is dry.

Among moisturizers, glycerol and urea (a natural component of NMF not related to filaggrin degradation products) are preferred. Both substances are physiological humectants that play a key role in maintaining the hydration of the *stratum corneum* (Giménez-Arnau A., 2016).

Urea is more effective than glycerol at low horny layer water content. Still, its physical properties (e.g., sensitivity to heat, pH dependence of structural stability, tendency to precipitate) can be problematic for emollient production. In addition, urea must dissolve to exert its effect, and it may not show its impact on a desiccated *stratum corneum*. When moisturizer is included as an emollient ingredient, it must be used at the optimal concentration. For example, if the formula contains too much glycerin, it will dry the skin due to its hygroscopic nature (Albèr C. et al., 2014).

Experts have also confirmed the significant role of dexpanthenol in the composition of topical emollients in the restoration of skin hydration. Among the numerous functions of dexpanthenol are the compensation of reduced hydration by increasing water content and its favorable effects on the molecular mobility/fluidity of lipid lamellae and the *stratum corneum* proteins. Another key feature of dexpanthenol is its beneficial effect on epidermal regeneration by enhancing epidermal differentiation. By supporting epidermal regeneration, dexpanthenol helps restore the barrier function in dry skin, promoting normal epidermal cell differentiation. The latter property addresses long-term dry skin problems and interrupts the dry skin cycle.

Since one of the main symptoms of AD is itching, emollients for dry atopic skin should contain an antipruritic/soothing agent.

Some emollients also include biologically active substances that are not classified as topical medicines and do not require a license. These are called "emollients plus" and may contain, for example, flavonoids such as licochalcone A, saponins, and riboflavin from protein-free oat germ extracts, bacterial lysates from *Aquaphilus dolomiae* or *Vitreoscilla filiformis* species, or a synthetic menthol derivative such as menthoxypropanediol (Wollenberg A. et al., 2018).

3.2.2. Recommendations for use

It is essential to choose the right type of emulsion (water-in-oil or oil-in-water) depending on the affected area of the body, the phase of the disease course (acute or chronic), the time of year, and the patient's skin characteristics.

Acute lesions generally require hydrophilic preparations, whereas chronic lesions necessitate lipophilic preparations. Lipophilic preparations should be used on extensor surfaces; flexor (inner surface of the fold) and intertriginous (areas where two areas may touch and rub against each other) zones should never be treated with overly oily substances. Hydrophilic preparations are preferred in summer and lipophilic preparations in winter. Sometimes, emollients are poorly tolerated when used in areas with a pronounced inflammatory response during AD exacerbations. In such cases, anti-inflammatory therapy should be performed first (Wollenberg A. et al., 2022).

However, the amount of emollient used is crucial for the success of topical basal therapy. The so-called fingertip unit (FTU) is defined as the amount of ointment, cream, or other semi-solid dosage form dispensed from a tube with a 5 mm nozzle and applied from the distal skin fold to the tip of an adult index finger (approximately 0.5 g) (**Fig. II-3-1**). This amount is sufficient to treat two adult palms. Effective AD therapy requires at least 250 g of emollient per week for a child and 500 g for an adult (Wollenberg A. et al., 2018).

Moreover, emollients should be applied immediately after bathing and gently drying the skin by blotting with a soft towel, as the effects of emollient application without bathing take longer to manifest (Chiang C., Eichenfield L.F., 2009).

Skin hydration is usually maintained by applying emollients with a hydrophilic base, such as 5% urea or glycerin, at least twice daily (Angelova-Fischer I. et al., 2018). Prolonged use of maintenance (e.g., twice-weekly) emollient therapy once remission has been attained may increase the duration of relapse-free intervals (Akerstrom U. et al., 2015).

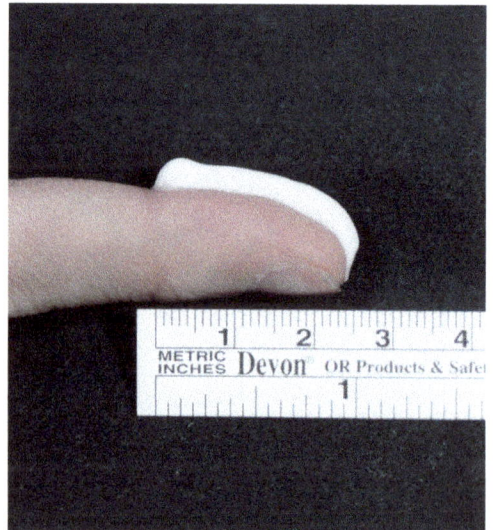

Figure II-3-1. Fingertip unit (FTU) (adapted from Kim J.E. et al., 2015)

3.3. What ingredients in cosmetic products should atopic patients be wary of?

Generally, any substance in a cosmetic product can be an allergen for a particular person. However, cosmetic ingredients differ in their allergenicity from low to high, depending on the frequency with which an adverse response occurs. This is especially true for patients with AD, in whom the epidermal barrier is impaired, and skin sensitivity to foreign agents is heightened.

These individuals (especially children under two years of age) should only use products that do not contain protein allergens or haptens* that cause contact allergy (Angelova-Fischer I. et al., 2018). In this section, we present substances to be avoided by atopic patients.

3.3.1. Ingredients of cosmetics with a high risk of skin sensitization

The Scientific Committee on Cosmetic Products and Non-food Products Intended for Consumers (SCCNFP) has approved the 7th amendment to EU Directive 76/768/EEC, Annex VIII, containing a list of 26 ingredients based on dermatological studies, which cosmetic manufacturers are obliged to list on the label of the final cosmetic product to protect consumers who are allergic or intolerant to a component of the registered substances. Including such chemicals in the list of ingredients on the label is mandatory if their concentration in the final product is 0.01% for products that wash off the skin surface and 0.001% for products that remain on the skin surface.

Preservatives, especially those that release formaldehyde, some UV filters, and fragrances, both natural (essential oils) and synthetic (**Table II-3-2**), are in the risk group. Not all these substances are allergens, but some (e.g., oxybenzone) increase skin sensitivity to sunlight and are classed as photosensitizers.

---

* Haptens are low-molecular-weight substances (up to 10 kDa) that do not possess antigenicity and acquire it by increasing their molecular weight (e.g., by attaching to a specific carrier protein). The carrier stimulates Th cells, which help B cells respond to hapten.

Table II-3-2. Some components of cosmetic products causing skin sensitization (according to the EU Cosmetics Directive 76/768/EEC). INCI — International Nomenclature of Cosmetic Ingredients

INCI	CHEMICAL NATURE	COMMENTS
2-Bromo-2-nitro-propane-1,3-diol DMDM hydantoin Imidazolidinyl urea Diazolidinyl urea Quaternium-15	Substances releasing formalde-hyde	Preservatives
Methylparaben Propylparaben	Parabens: methyl-4-hydroxy-benzoate and propyl-4-hydroxy-benzoate	Preservatives
Methylchloroiso-thiazolinone (and) methyliso-thiazolinone	A mixture of two preservatives	A preservative acceptable for use in products that need to be rinsed off, such as shampoos
Parfume	Fragrances (synthetic and in es-sential oils)	Giving the body a pleas-ant odor
Lanolin and lano-lin derivatives	Lanolin (wool wax, animal wax) is a mixture of esters of high-molecular-weight alcohols (cholesterol, isocholesterol, etc.) with higher fatty acids (myristic, palmitic, cerotinic, etc.) and free high-molecular-weight alcohols	Softening ingredient
Colophonium	Rosin gum (Greek pitch, *Pix graeca*) is a solid constituent of resinous substances of coniferous trees, remaining after distillation of volatile substances from them. It contains 60–92% of resin acids (mainly abietinic), 0.5–12% of saturated and unsaturated fatty acids, and 8–20% of neutral substances (sesqui-, di-, and triterpenoids)	Pine resin of A Grade is used in lipsticks, nail varnishes, and varnish-pastes in concentrations up to 4.0%

Continued on p. 107

INCI	CHEMICAL NATURE	COMMENTS
Tosylamide/ formaldehyde resin	Tosylamide/formaldehyde resin	Included in the base of nail polish, releases formaldehyde
p-Phenylenedi-amine p-Toluenediamine	Para-phenylenediamine Para-toluenediamine	Hair dyes
Butylhydroxytolu-ene (BHT)	Butylhydroxytoluene, ionol	Lipophilic antioxidant, synthetic "analog" of vitamin E, also used as a food preservative
Benzophenone-3	Oxybenzone	UVA/B filter, in concentrations greater than 0.5% may increase skin sensitivity to sunlight (photosensitization)
Butyl methoxydibenzoyl methane	Avobenzone	Fat-soluble UVA filter, rapidly degrades when exposed to light, so it is necessary to stabilize it (e.g., with octocrylene, cyclodextrins, etc.)
Octyl dimethyl PABA	A derivative of para-aminoben-zoic acid	UVB filter, may cause contact dermatitis or increase skin sensitivity to sunlight (photosensitization)
Ethylhexyl methoxycinna-mate	Cinnamic acid derivative	UVB filter, fat-soluble, maximum permissible concentration of 7.5%
Resorcinol	Dihydroxybenzene, resorcinol	Used as an antiseptic and disinfectant at a 5–10% concentration in oil-based shampoos, anti-dandruff shampoos, and photoprotective skincare products, and together with lactic and salicylic acids in Jessner's solution for chemical peels

3.3.2. Fragrances

Fragrance compounds are the most allergenic. Most cosmetic formulations denote them as perfume or fragrance, which is wrong from a dermatological point of view because fragrances differ in their chemical nature and degree of danger to the skin.

According to the current EU Cosmetics Directive 76/768/EEC, fragrance substances must be provided separately in the ingredients list if their concentration exceeds 0.001% in preparations that remain on the skin for a long time and 0.01% in washed-off products. Such substances include (International Nomenclature of Cosmetic Ingredients — INCI names):

- alpha-Isomethyl ionone
- Amyl cinnamal
- Amylcinnamyl alcohol
- Anise alcohol
- Benzyl alcohol
- Benzyl benzoate
- Benzyl cinnamate
- Benzyl salicylate
- Butylphenyl methylpropional
- Cinnamal
- Cinnamyl alcohol
- Citral
- Citronellol
- Coumarin
- Eugenol
- *Evernia prunastri, Evernia furfuracea*
- Farnesol
- Geraniol
- Hexyl cinnamal
- Hydroxycitronellal
- Hydroxyisohexyl 3-cyclohexene carboxaldehyde
- Isoeugenol
- Limonene
- Linalool
- Methyl 2-octynoate

3.3.3. Nut extracts

Those with food allergies to nuts should avoid cosmetics containing nut extracts. **Table II-3-3** lists the most common nuts with their Latin names (also used in the INCI) and their common names in English. To determine the degree of allergenicity of a particular ingredient, a repeated patch test is used: occlusive patches with the substance in question are first applied to 50–200 participants, and, after a rest period, the substance is applied again, but on a different skin area.

Table II-3-3. Nut sources of cosmetic ingredients

INCI / LATIN NAME	COMMON NAME
Prunus amygdalus Prunus amara	Almond Bitter almond
Prunus dulcis	Sweet almond
Bertholletia excelsa	Brazil nut
Anacardium occidentale	Cashew nut
Castanea sativa	Chestnut
Cocos nucifera*	Coconut*
Corylus avellana Corylus americana Corylus rostrata	Hazelnut
Aesculus hippocastanum	Horse chestnut
Cola vera	Kola nut
Aleurites muluccana	Kukui nut
Macadamia ternifolia Macadamia integrifolia	Macadamia nut
Arachis hypogaea	Peanut
Pistacia vera Pistacia lentiscus	Pistachio nut
Juglans regia Juglans mandshurica Juglans nigra	Walnut
Sesamum indicum	Sesame seed

* Coconut very rarely causes food allergies.

Chapter 4
Nutrition and nutraceutical support

4.1. Food allergy in adult atopic patients

AD may first occur in adulthood or be an extension of the pediatric form of the disease, which is often seen in patients with severe pediatric AD and respiratory manifestations of allergy.

The prevalence of AD in adults generally ranges from 1 to 3% according to different estimates (in comparison, in children, it is up to 20%). In adults, as in children, clear associations with other atopic diseases, including allergic rhinitis and asthma, have been described. While IgE-mediated food allergy, such as to eggs, cow's milk, and peanuts, is a characteristic and widespread factor in atopic dermatitis in children, the relationship between food sensitization, clinical food allergy, and AD in adults remains poorly understood.

Schafer T. et al. (2001) evaluated the incidence of AD among 1,537 adult patients (aged 25–74) with food allergies (defined as a history of symptoms of an immediate allergic reaction to foods, with cutaneous manifestations), 10.1% of whom had AD. Considering that the prevalence of AD in the general population averages at about 2%, it appears that food allergies are, on average, five times more common among adults with AD than among those without AD.

On the other hand, Celakovska J. et al. (2011a, 2011b, 2012) studied the prevalence of food allergy to wheat, eggs, and cow's milk in 179 atopic patients aged 14–63 years. All patients underwent the following diagnostic procedures:

- Food provocation (ingestion of certain foods with the subsequent recording of clinical symptoms of allergy) using the most common food allergens — eggs, cow's milk, and wheat
- Scarification skin test (drops of solutions with food allergens are applied to the skin of the forearm, then through the drops of solutions, the skin is pricked with a special scarifier, and the skin reaction to the allergen is subsequently studied)
- Serum test for specific IgE*

All patients were monitored for 12 months, and the dynamics of AD symptoms with and without an elimination diet were evaluated. Food allergy symptoms were rare during food provocation, whereas laboratory tests documented more frequent allergic sensitization to food allergens (**Table II-4-1**).

Table II-4-1. Comparison of laboratory markers and clinical manifestations of food allergy in adult atopic patients (Celakovska J. et al., 2011a, 2011b, 2012)

FOOD ALLERGEN	CLINICAL MANIFESTATIONS OF FOOD ALLERGY CAUSED BY FOOD PROVOCATION	ELEVATION OF SPECIFIC IgE
Wheat	4.5%	11.2%
Egg	6.1%	28%
Cow's milk	0.6%	9.5%

Only 50% of patients with clinical symptoms of food allergy improved by following the elimination diet. On the other hand, even in the presence of laboratory signs of immune system hypersensitivity to food allergens, clinical manifestations were observed 2.5–16 times less frequently, depending on the allergen.

---

* Immunoglobulin E (IgE) is a class of immunoglobulins synthesized mainly by plasma cells of mucous membranes. The primary biological role of IgE is its unique ability to bind to the surface of human mast cells and basophils. Degranulation of mast cells and basophils "turns on" the sequential events leading to the release of inflammatory mediators — the allergic response. For this reason, IgE has been selected as a marker of allergy.

These findings suggest that, in adult patients, food allergies characteristic of childhood AD recede into the background. Within the atopic march*, a more pronounced immune system response to aeroallergens is observed. Birch pollen allergy may present a different clinical scenario: in the presence of sensitization to birch pollen, the immune system begins to react to similar food allergens such as apples, peaches, cherries, plums, apricots, carrots, celery, zucchini, legumes, and nuts.

Werfel T. et al. (1999) studied the role of foods with antigen structure similarities to birch pollen (carrot, celery, hazelnut, and apple) in atopic patients aged 17–64 years with severe sensitization to birch pollen (specific IgE > 17.5 kU/l) without a history of food allergy. All 37 patients were on an elimination diet to avoid all birch pollen-associated foods and were monitored on an outpatient basis before undergoing food provocation testing with carrots, celery, hazelnuts, and apples. In 17 cases (45.9%), an exacerbation of AD during the food provocation was noted, with an increase in severity of at least 15 points from baseline on the SCORAD, which serves as a tool for an objective assessment of AD severity. In addition, significantly higher levels of specific IgE to food close in antigenicity to birch pollen were found in patients with a marked reaction to food provocation.

These findings indicate that the exacerbation of AD caused by pollen-related cross-allergens should be considered in adult atopic patients.

4.2. Nutraceutical support

Evidence suggests that diet-related factors, including body weight, fatty acid intake, and consumption of foods with pro-inflammatory properties, among others, may influence the clinical manifestations of AD.

---

* Atopic march is a phenomenon in which some allergic diseases progress to more serious ones or lead to the development of others. The debut of the march is the peak of food allergies, which usually occurs in the first year of a child's life. Later in life, the allergy moves to another target organ — the respiratory tract. Sensitivity to respiratory allergens — pollen, house dust mites, fungal spores — is added to food allergies. Seasonal or year-round allergic rhinitis may eventually develop into bronchial asthma.

Maintaining a healthy weight

Obesity and AD share pathologic features such as insulin resistance, leptin resistance, and inflammation. Increasing evidence indicates that obesity predisposes a person to develop and/or worsen AD, while AD increases the risk of obesity. Cytokines, chemokines, and immune cells mediate this correlation. Obese individuals with AD are more resistant to anti-inflammatory therapy. At the same time, weight loss may alleviate the AD course. Effective AD treatment and weight loss can improve the well-being of people with both diseases (Yang S. et al., 2023).

Food rationing

According to the findings of the Korean National Health and Nutrition Study, which involved 17,000 participants, the risk of developing AD was 57% higher in people whose diets included a high proportion of meat and chemically and thermally processed foods (the so-called Western diet) (**Fig. II-4-1**) (Park S. et al., 2016).

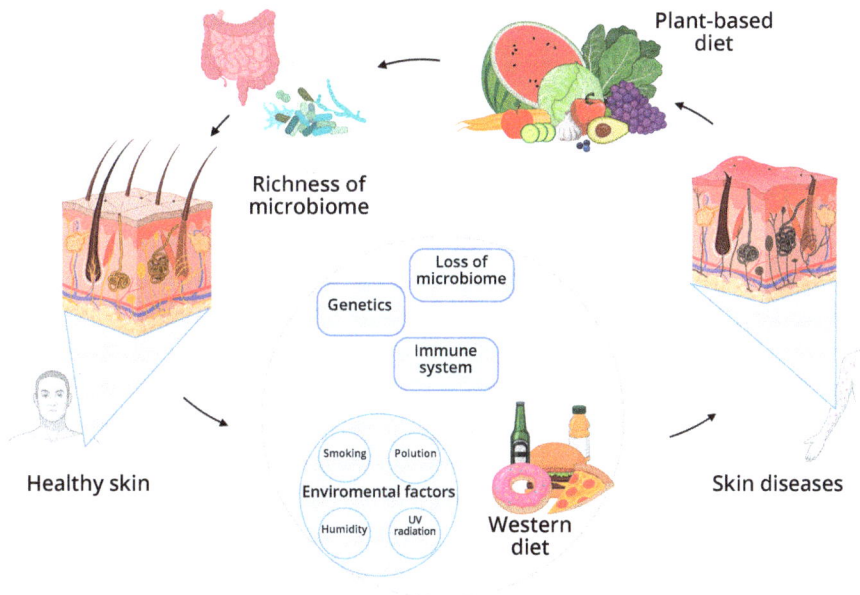

Figure II-4-1. Effect of Western diet on skin health (adapted from Flores-Balderas X. et al., 2023)

Western diet

Plant-based diets

Dietary patterns

Gut-microbiome axis

Skin effects

Dysregulation of microbiota

Improve of microbiota

Elasticity
Firmness
Depigmentation

Elasticity
Firmness
Depigmentation

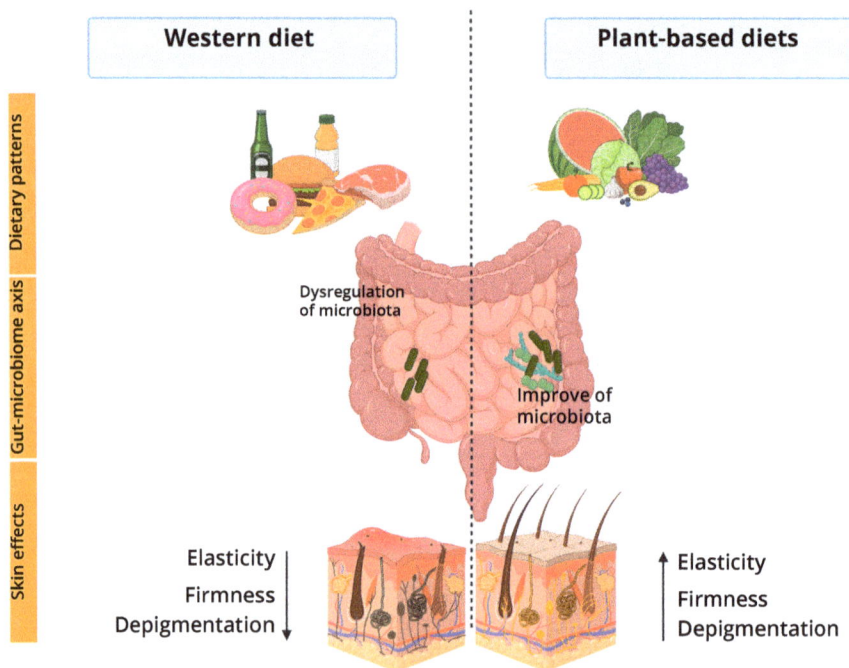

Figure II-4-2. Improvements of the skin's structural and functional status due to a plant-based diet (adapted from Flores-Balderas X. et al., 2023)

According to the International Study of Asthma and Allergy in Childhood (ISAAC), a diet mostly comprising fresh fruits and legumes was associated with a 40% reduction in AD risk (Cepeda A.M. et al., 2015).

Generally, a plant-based diet is beneficial for skin health as it helps modulate inflammatory and oxidative processes, which are the main mechanisms of the pathogenesis of inflammatory dermatoses (**Fig. II-4-2**) (Flores-Balderas X. et al., 2023). Yet, there is no consensus regarding its influence on AD. While no relationship between a plant-based diet and clinical manifestations of AD was found in some studies (Zhang J. et al., 2022), other data suggest that a vegetarian diet reduces the severity of AD symptoms as measured by the SCORAD scale. This improvement seems to be related to a decrease in the levels of eosinophils and neutrophils in the circulating blood and a decrease in monocyte production of prostaglandin E2, which activates Th2 cells and IgE production (Tanaka T. et al., 2001). A low-calorie diet (55% of the estimated energy requirement) has also been found to to exert positive effect on the health status of atopic patients (Kouda K. et al., 2000).

Fatty acids in foods — mainly unsaturated fatty acids, which are components of cell membranes and precursors of immunomodulators — also seem to play a role in the pathogenesis of some AD symptoms. Since the human body cannot synthesize them, fatty acids must be obtained from the diet in the form of so-called exogenous fatty acids: linoleic acid (precursor of arachidonic acid) and α-linolenic acid — the precursor of eicosapentaenoic acid (EPA) and docosahexaenoic acid (DHA). Their deficiency contributes to the development of certain diseases, such as the cardiovascular or nervous system, or exacerbates disease course/symptoms, such as skin itching and dryness in atopic dermatitis. Although the available clinical studies support the efficacy of fatty acid supplementation in AD treatment, their results are not unequivocal (Kaczmarski M. et al., 2013). In a systematic review and meta-analysis of studies on the effects of fish consumption or fish oil supplementation, their high proportion in the diet was associated with a reduced AD incidence by almost 50% compared to low fish consumption or placebo (Best K.P. et al., 2016).

4.3. Vitamin D and atopic dermatitis

Although the evidence for the benefits of vitamin D supplementation is mixed, in specific patient populations, particularly those with low baseline vitamin D levels and frequent skin infections, vitamin D supplementation may benefit AD (Best K.P. et al., 2016).

Vitamin D enters the body with some foods and is synthesized in the skin. Irrespective of its entry route, vitamin D is biologically inert, requiring conversion in the body for activation. The first step of activation occurs in the liver, where vitamin D is converted to hydroxyvitamin D (25(OH)D; calcifediol, calcidiol), and the second step occurs in the kidneys to form the active form 1,25-dihydroxyvitamin D (1,25(OH)$_2$D; also known as calcitriol). The complete cycle of formation of the active vitamin D form can occur in the epidermis in keratinocytes, where calcitriol synthesis is carried out, bypassing the liver and kidneys. These are the only cells in the body with a complete calcitriol synthesis cycle (Slominski A.T. et al., 2015).

The primary function of vitamin D is to regulate calcium and phosphorus metabolism, but its spectrum of action is much broader. Like other steroid hormones, the active form of vitamin D binds to its receptor — vitamin D receptor (VDR), which forms a heterodimer with the retinoid X receptor (RXR) that affects the expression of more than 900 genes, which is equivalent to 3–5% of the entire human genome (Ombra M.N. et al., 2017). VDRs regulate gene expression in cell proliferation, differentiation, cell detoxification metabolism, ion transport across the cell membrane, cellular senescence, and apoptosis. In addition, calcitriol improves DNA repair, enhances defense against reactive oxygen species (ROS), and has an immunomodulatory effect.

Calcitriol affects several hundred genes regulating innate and acquired immunity through its receptors. Vitamin D:

- Participates in the body's nonspecific response to pathogens and tissue damage through stimulation of monocyte differentiation into mature macrophages
- Enhances the production of antimicrobial peptides through stimulation of toll-like receptors (TLRs)
- Inhibits differentiation, maturation, and immunostimulatory capacity of dendritic cells
- Stimulates the production of IL-10 and other anti-inflammatory cytokines by regulatory T cells and reduces the secretion of pro-inflammatory cytokines
- Inhibits immunoglobulin release and initiates apoptosis in B cells, which produce autoantibodies

4.3.1. Dermatologic aspects of vitamin D status

Vitamin D synthesized in keratinocytes, in turn, protects them from the harmful effects of UV radiation, reducing the number of cells in a state of apoptosis after irradiation. The protective effect is evidenced by increased expression of the p53 protein, which facilitates DNA repair. Vitamin D also helps to avoid DNA damage caused by nitric oxide products and inhibits UV-induced immunosuppression (Dixon K.M. et al., 2013).

Sunscreen use reduces vitamin D production by 83–92.5% (depending on the degree of protection). Still, it has almost no effect on vitamin D levels in the blood, which Libon F. et al. (2017) ascribe to the body's capacity to switch to endogenous sources of vitamin D precursors.

4.3.2. Blood vitamin D levels in atopic dermatitis

Vitamin D deficiency in pregnant women affects the development of the fetal immune system and immune regulation in early childhood. A cohort study of 763 Japanese mother–child dyads showed that the risk of AD and respiratory allergic manifestations was significantly reduced among children aged 16–24 months whose mothers took vitamin D supplements during pregnancy (Miyake Y. et al., 2010).

A meta-analysis conducted by Hattangdi-Haridas S.R. et al. (2019) showed a decrease in vitamin D levels by an average of 14 nmol/l in adults and 16 nmol/l in children with AD, as well as the effect of blood vitamin D levels on the SCORAD index. In a more recent study, the relationship between vitamin D levels, eosinophils, and severity of AD manifestations according to the SCORAD was evaluated more thoroughly (Çiçek F., Köle M.T., 2023). The authors found that serum vitamin D level and eosinophil count significantly influenced the SCORAD index. Specifically, for every unit increase in serum vitamin D level, the SCORAD index decreased by 0.449. Similarly, an increase in eosinophils by one unit led to a 0.009 rise in the SCORAD index. It is worth noting that the effect of serum vitamin D level on disease severity was superior to that of eosinophil count. The authors found a negative relationship between serum vitamin D levels and the SCORAD index: lower vitamin D levels corresponded to higher SCORAD values and more severe AD.

4.3.3. Use of vitamin D in atopic dermatitis

Maintaining optimal vitamin D levels prevents allergic diseases, including AD, and contributes to their favorable course and improved prognosis.

Including vitamin D in the treatment (1,500–1,600 IU/day) was found by Hattangdi-Haridas S.R. et al. (2019) to positively affect secondary rash infection, IgE levels, and total eosinophil count.

A significant reduction in *S. aureus* colonization, SCORAD index, and erythema severity was also observed by the 4th week of vitamin D treatment in 20 patients who took part in the Udompataikul M. et al.'s (2015) study. Still, the treatment did not affect itching, dryness, lichenification, and skin hydration. A positive effect of vitamin D supplementation was observed in 11 children from Boston, USA, with winter exacerbation of AD (Sidbury R. et al., 2008) and 104 children from Mongolia (Camargo C.A. et al., 2014).

According to Umehara Y. et al. (2023), vitamin D can also be a topical therapy for AD. Following topical calcitriol applications to the skin of mice with induced AD, the authors found the following positive effects of vitamin D on the structural and functional state of the skin compared to untreated mice:

- Reduction in the AD severity scores
- Reduction in the epidermis thickness
- Improvement of the barrier function of the *stratum corneum* according to TEWL and the number of tight junctions (**Fig. II-4-3**)
- Decreased expression of pro-inflammatory cytokines such as IL-13 and IL-33

These results suggest that topical application of calcitriol may improve AD symptoms by restoring the epidermal barrier.

4.3.4. Correction of vitamin D insufficiency and deficiency

Vitamin D content in the blood of 20–29 ng/ml signifies insufficiency, while levels below 20 ng/ml indicate vitamin D deficiency.

Almost all medications intended to correct vitamin D levels in the blood contain cholecalciferol (D3), which can be administered in solutions or capsules. The dose depends on the vitamin D serum level.

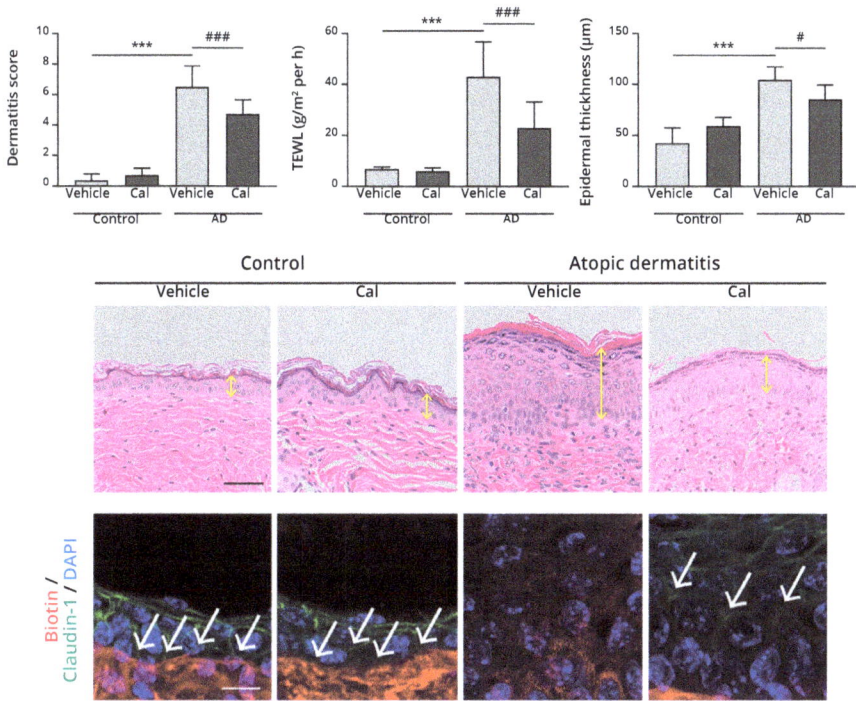

Figure II-4-3. Reduction in the severity of AD symptoms in mice after topical application of calcitriol (Cal) (adapted from Umehara Y. et al., 2023)

Immunofluorescence was used to estimate the number of tight junctions. The protein of tight junctions, claudin, is colored green, and the indicator substance, biotin, is colored red. Arrows indicate areas of tight junctions that prevent the passage of the indicator.

After the COVID-19 pandemic, recommendations for vitamin D intake for prophylactic and therapeutic purposes were adjusted, as summarized below (Bleizgys A., 2021).

Prophylactic use

■ The following daily dose is recommended to maintain normal levels of vitamin D:
  – Infants (<6 months): 400–600 IU
  – Children (1–10 years): 600–1,000 IU
  – Adolescents (11–18 years): 800–2,000 IU
  – Adults (18–75 years): 1,000–2,000 IU
  – Elderly (≥75 years): 2,000–4,000 IU

- For individuals at risk (e.g., due to obesity, malabsorption, renal disease, etc.), the dose can be increased by 2–3 times
- The maximum safe dose is 10,000 IU/day

Therapeutic administration (for vitamin D deficiency)
- When 25(OH)D levels are below 25 nmol/l:
  - Children (1–10 years): 3,000–6,000 IU/day for three months
  - Adolescents and adults: 6,000 IU/day or 50,000 IU/week for 2–3 months
- At 25(OH)D levels of 25–75 nmol/l:
  - Increasing the current dose by 1.5–2 times or taking the maximum prophylactic dose for a given age for 2–3 months

General recommendations
- Determining 25(OH)D in the blood before administering it is advisable. If such analysis cannot be performed, it is recommended to start with a dose of 4,000 IU/day with subsequent testing after 1–1.5 months
- Patients at risk of hypercalcemia (e.g., those with granulomatous diseases) require individualized dose adjustment and regular monitoring of calcium levels

Factors influencing efficacy
- Adherence to the recommendations for intake and course duration
- Presence of chronic diseases, malabsorption, or calcium and magnesium deficiencies that may interfere with normal vitamin D levels
- In complicated cases, a more bioavailable form of vitamin D, such as calcidiol, may be preferable

By following these guidelines, vitamin D levels can be effectively maintained and restored, improving overall health.

Attention! Vitamin D in the blood should be monitored every 6–12 months.

Food allergy in adult atopic patients occurs less frequently than in children and adolescents and is characterized by milder symptoms. Nevertheless, the risk of food allergy in AD remains higher than in the general population. On the other hand, adult atopic patients may unnecessarily avoid potentially allergenic foods or those that caused them allergies in childhood, such as dairy, seafood, nuts, and cereals, which can lead to nutritional deficiencies and exacerbate barrier function disorders characteristic of atopic skin. A possible compromise may be a reasonable **elimination diet** — exclusion from the diet of a particular food product at high levels of specific IgE accompanied by clinical symptoms of food allergy (Guibas G.V. et al., 2013). Such issues should never be solved without consulting an allergist.

In adulthood, the focus should shift to the next stage of the atopic march: respiratory allergic manifestations, especially hypersensitivity to birch pollen and cross-antigens characteristic of this condition. **During the period of increased birch pollen concentration in the air, AD patients should limit their consumption of fruits, vegetables, legumes, and nuts.**

4.4. The use of probiotics in atopic dermatitis

The communities of microorganisms living in the gut and the skin perform essential health maintenance functions. The contribution of changes in the species composition of the gut microbiome to the development of inflammatory skin diseases is an undeniable fact confirmed by long-term studies (Koh L.F. et al., 2022).

4.4.1. Systemic administration of probiotics

The gut microbiome has a modulating effect on the human immune system. Disruption of the optimal species composition in the microbiome can trigger autoimmune reactions and lead to an inflammatory response at the gut and skin level (Szántó M. et al., 2019). The immune

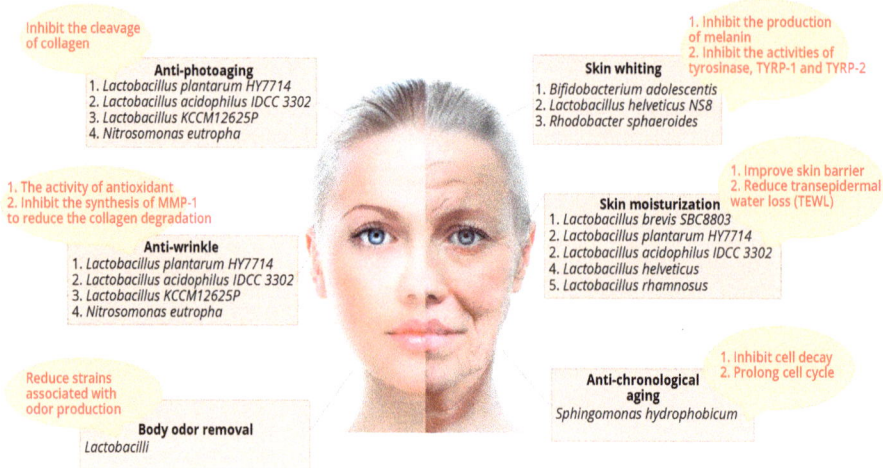

Figure II-4-4. The skin improvement effect of probiotics and its related mechanism (adapted from Gao T. et al., 2023)

The skin-improving effects of probiotics include anti-photoaging (collagen cleavage inhibition), skin whitening (inhibit the production of melanin and the activity of tyrosinase, TYRP-1, and TYRP-2), anti-wrinkle (antioxidant activity and inhibition of the synthesis of matrix metalloproteinase-1 — MMP-1 — to reduce the degradation of collagen), skin moisturization (improve skin barrier and reduce TEWL), body odor removal (reduced abundance of strains associated with odor production), and anti-chronological aging (inhibit cell decay and prolong cell cycle).

system seems to serve as a link between the skin and the gut. The interaction between the microbiome and the host immune systems is vital in maintaining skin homeostasis (De Pessemier B. et al., 2021). The gut–skin axis suggests a relationship in which the modulating influence of the microbiome on the immune system can be utilized to improve skin health (**Fig. II-4-4**). Shaping a healthy skin or gut microbiome composition with systemic probiotics is a potential clinical approach to treating inflammatory dermatoses, including AD and psoriasis (**Fig. II-4-5**).

The mechanisms by which the gut microbiome influences skin condition in AD are discussed below.

Immunologic pathway

When taken orally, probiotics can interact with the gastrointestinal mucosa and gut-associated lymphoid tissue (GALT), which includes

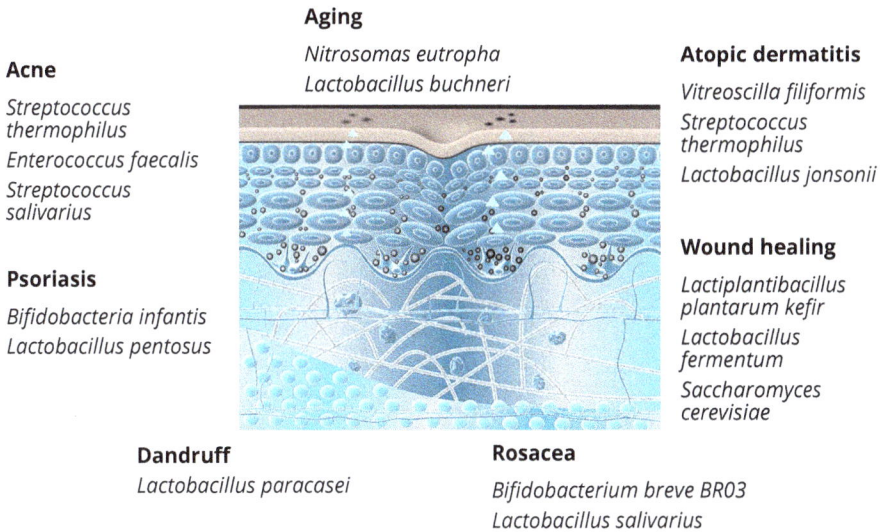

Aging

Nitrosomas eutropha
Lactobacillus buchneri

Acne

Streptococcus thermophilus
Enterococcus faecalis
Streptococcus salivarius

Atopic dermatitis

Vitreoscilla filiformis
Streptococcus thermophilus
Lactobacillus jonsonii

Psoriasis

Bifidobacteria infantis
Lactobacillus pentosus

Wound healing

Lactiplantibacillus plantarum kefir
Lactobacillus fermentum
Saccharomyces cerevisiae

Dandruff

Lactobacillus paracasei

Rosacea

Bifidobacterium breve BR03
Lactobacillus salivarius

Figure II-4-5. Probiotics used in the treatment of skin diseases (adapted from Gao T. et al., 2023)

Different probiotics can be used to treat various skin diseases. For example, *Nitrosomonas eutropha* and *Lactobacillus buchneri* can improve skin aging; *Streptococcus thermophiles*, *Enterococcus faecalis*, and *Streptococcus salivarius* can improve acne; *Vitreoscilla filiformis*, *Streptococcus thermophilus*, and *Lactobacillus johnsonii* can improve atopic dermatitis; *Bifidobacteria infantis* and *Lactobacillus pentosus* can improve psoriasis; *Lactiplantibacillus plantarum kefir*, *Lactobacillus fermentum*, and *Saccharomyces cerevisiae* can improve wound healing; *Lactobacillus paracasei* can improve dandruff; *Bifidobacterium breve BR03* and *Lactobacillus salivarius* can improve rosacea.

more than 70% of immune system cells (Lebeer S. et al., 2010). Probiotics stimulate an increase in the number of regulatory T lymphocytes that control the strength and duration of the immune response, inhibit the synthesis of pro-inflammatory cytokines (IL-4, IL-17, INF-γ), and increase the level of anti-inflammatory cytokines (IL-10, TGF-β, TNFβ) (**Fig. II-4-6**) (Kim H.J. et al., 2013; Chang Y. et al., 2016).

Metabolite pathway

Metabolites produced by the gut microbiome, including SCFAs, also link the gut and the skin. SCFAs produced by gut bacteria have a meaningful impact on AD etiopathogenesis, which may be explained by the relationship with skin immunity. As a part of their study, Kaikiri H. et al. (2017) showed that linoleic acid and 10-hydroxy-*cis*-12-octadecenoic acid

Effect of pre/probiotics in AD

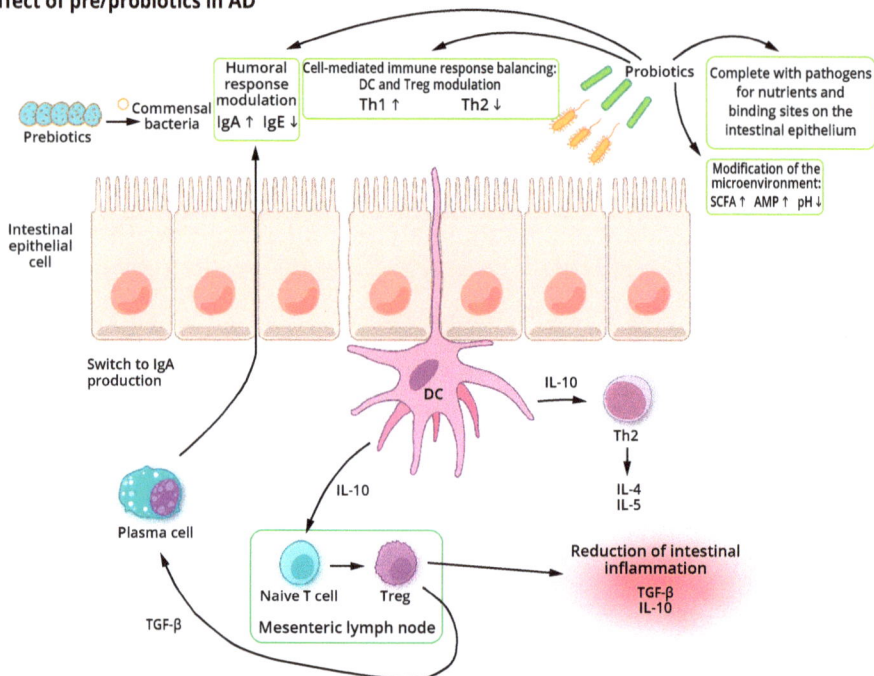

Figure II-4-6. Immune mechanisms of prebiotics and probiotics (adapted from Kim J.E., Kim H.S., 2019)

Prebiotics feed the commensal bacteria and probiotics. Probiotics modulate the humoral response (an increase in IgA and a decrease in IgE levels), balance cell-mediated immune response (an increase in Treg number and a decrease in Th2 response), compete with pathogens, and modify the microenvironment. SCFA — short-chain fatty acid; AMP — anti-microbial peptide; DC — dendritic cell; IL — interleukin; TGF — tumor growth factor; IgE — immunoglobulin E; IgA — immunoglobulin A; Th1 — T helper 1 cells; Th2 — T helper 2 cells.

alleviate the AD course and control the gut microbiome composition in mice. The role of three differentiated subgroups of the neonatal gut microbiota (NGM1–3) and its metabolites in early allergic sensitization has also been identified (Johnson A.M.F., DePaolo R.W., 2017). Among these three subgroups, NGM3 is associated with multiple allergic sensitizations. The proportion of *Bifidobacterium*, *Ackermannia*, and *Fasciola* in its composition was relatively low. Moreover, according to the *in vitro* study conducted by Gao T. et al. (2023), 12,13-dihydroxy-9-octadecenoic acid (12,13-diHome) — a metabolite with pro-inflammatory effects — was abundant in NGM3. Besides, the content of 12,13-diHome

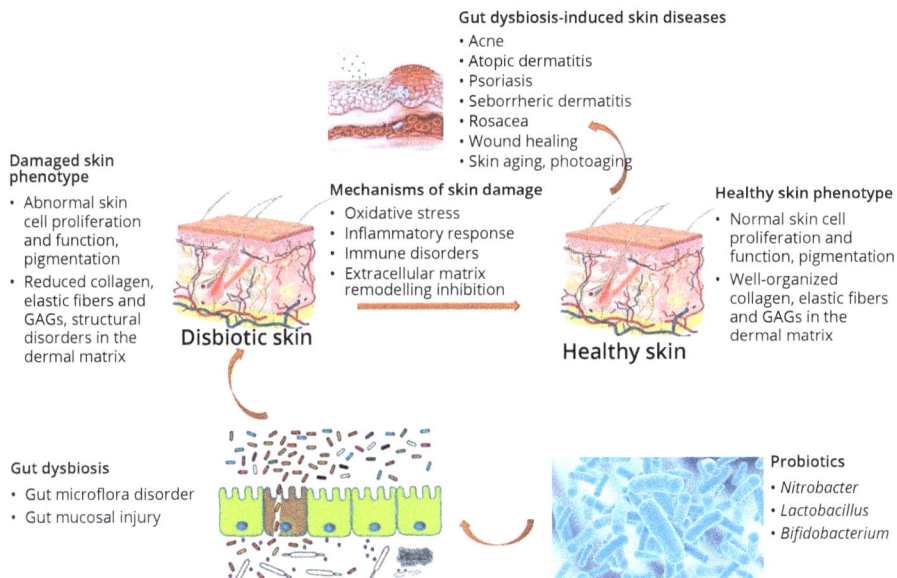

Figure II-4-7. The mechanism by which probiotics improve the symptoms of skin diseases (adapted from Gao T. et al., 2023)

Probiotics, including *Nitrobacter*, *Lactobacillus*, and *Bifidobacterium*, can restore intestinal homeostasis by improving intestinal microbiota disorders and repairing intestinal mucosal damage. They can also be used to treat skin damage phenotype, including abnormal skin cell proliferation and function, pigmentation, reduced collagen, elastic fibers, glycosaminoglycan (GAG), and structural disorders in the dermis by inhibiting oxidative stress, inflammation response, immune homeostasis, and extracellular matrix (ECM) remodeling inhibition, ultimately helping counteract chronic inflammatory dermatoses (acne, atopic dermatitis, psoriasis, seborrheic dermatitis, and rosacea) as well as photoaging and aging skin, while promoting wound healing.

was elevated in the protective layer of vernix caseosa — the white waxy plaque on the skin of newborns. These results point to the likely contribution of the metabolite pathway to the interaction along the gut–skin axis (**Fig. II-4-7**).

Neuroendocrine pathway

The skin and gut microbiomes can interact through neuroendocrine signaling. This influence can be realized directly or indirectly (Yokoyama S. et al., 2015). Tryptophan production by intestinal microorganisms, which causes skin itching in atopic patients, is an example of direct signaling. Conversely, γ-aminobutyric acid produced by *Lactobacillus* and *Bifidobacterium* in the gut suppresses the skin itch.

Indirectly, intestinal commensals control serum levels of cytokines such as IL-10 and IFN-γ, which can lead to functional changes in the brain (Yokoyama S. et al., 2015). Cortisol is a stress hormone that can alter the permeability and barrier function of the intestinal epithelium by affecting the composition of the gut microbiome. Cortisol also alters the content of circulating neuroendocrine molecules, including tryptamine, trimethylamine, and 5-hydroxytryptamine, further enhancing the skin barrier and immune defense (Gao T. et al., 2023).

Probiotics are the most effective means of building a healthy gut and skin microbiome. The term "probiotic" means "for life" in Latin. Modern probiotics are live microorganisms that, when introduced in the required amount in food products, positively affect the gut microflora. Microorganisms belonging to the probiotic group are listed in **Table II-4-2**.

Table II-4-2. Microorganisms with probiotic properties (Lew L.C., Liong M.T., 2013)

LACTOBACILLUS	BIFIDO-BACTERIUM	ENTEROCOCCI	STREPTOCOCCI
Lact. acidophilus	Bif. adolescentis	Ent. faecalis	Strep. thermophilus
Lact. brevis	Bif. animalis	Ent. faecium	
Lact. casei	Bif. breve		
Lact. curvatus	Bif. infantis		
Lact. fermentum	Bif. longum		
Lact. gasseri	Bif. thermophilum		
Lact. johnsonii			
Lact. reuteri			
Lact. rhamnosus			
Lact. salivarius			
LACTOCOCCI	**PROPIONI-BACTERIUM**	**YEAST STRAINS**	**OTHERS**
L. lactis subsp. cremoris	P. freudenreichii	Kluyveromyces lactis	Leuconostoc mesenteroides
L. lactis subsp. lactis	P. freudenreichii subsp. shermanii	Saccharomyces boulardii	Pediococcus acidilactici
	P. jensenii	Saccharomyces cerevisiae	

Table II-4-3 summarizes the results of laboratory and clinical studies on using probiotics in atopic patients and experimental models of AD.

Table II-4-3. Efficacy of probiotics in atopic dermatitis: a review of laboratory and clinical studies

STUDY	PROBIOTIC STRAIN	RESULTS
Laboratory tests		
Won T.J. et al. (2011)	*Lactobacillus plantarum* *Lactobacillus rhamnosus*	Administration of *Lactobacillus plantarum* to mice resulted in regression of dermatitis induced by house dust mite antigens by increasing IL-10 production and altering the Th1/Th2-lymphocyte balance. After addition of *Lactobacillus rhamnosus*, suppression of mast cell-mediated inflammation was observed in the same mouse model.
Kim H.J. et al. (2013)	*Lactobacillus rhamnosus*	Oral administration of *Lactobacillus rhamnosus* to mice with induced AD was accompanied by increased levels of regulatory T cells and decreased levels of IL-4 and thymus stromal lymphopoietin.
Kim W.K. et al. (2021)	*Lactobacillus fermentum*	Oral administration of *Lactobacillus fermentum* to mice with induced AD was accompanied by clinical improvement, decreased serum IgE levels, decreased IL-4, -5, -13, and -31 levels, and increased anti-inflammatory cytokine IL-10 and TGF-β levels in the skin.
Clinical trials		
Di Marzio L. et al. (2003)	*Streptococcus thermophilus*	Improvement of structural and functional state of the *stratum corneum* by increasing the ceramide level in the skin in patients with AD.
Abrahamsson T.R. et al. (2007)	*Lactobacillus reuteri*	Administration of the probiotic *L. reuteri* reduces the incidence of IgE-dependent eczema in children.

Continued on p. 128

STUDY	PROBIOTIC STRAIN	RESULTS
Kukkonen K. et al. (2007)	*L. rhamnosus GG, L. rhamnosus LC705, B. breve Bb99,* and *Propionibacterium freudenreichii ssp. shermanii JS*	A sample comprising 1,223 pregnant women carrying children at high risk of allergy took placebo or probiotic capsules for 2–4 weeks. The newborns received the same capsules but with the prebiotic galacto-oligosaccharides or placebo for 6 months. Comparative analysis showed that the incidence of atopic eczema was significantly reduced in the experimental group.
Di Marzio L. et al. (2008)	*Streptococcus thermophilus*	Reducing the severity of eczema in atopic dermatitis, as well as the severity of other symptoms.
Drago L. et al. (2011) Matsumoto M. et al. (2014)	*B. animalis subsp. lactis* *L. acidophilus* *L. salivarius*	Regression of rashes was observed in patients taking probiotic strains.
Inoue Y. et al. (2015)	*Bifidobacterium bifidum* *Bifidobacterium lactis* *Lactobacillus acidophilus*	Pregnant women with a family history of AD received probiotics in the last four weeks of gestation, which were also given to their newborns during the first two months of life. The incidence of AD was significantly lower in the group receiving probiotics compared to the control group.
Kwon M.S. et al. (2018)	*Lactobacillus sakei*	Regression of rashes, decreased levels of CD^{4+} T and B cells, IgE, and Th2-cytokines in serum, along with an increase in the number of beneficial intestinal bacteria.
Jeong K. et al. (2020)	*Lactobacillus rhamnosus*	Probiotic administration once daily for 12 weeks to children with AD aged 1–12 years resulted in a reduction in the severity of clinical symptoms of the disease according to the SCORAD, as well as a decrease in eosinophil cationic protein and IL-31 levels.

Continued on p. 129

STUDY	PROBIOTIC STRAIN	RESULTS
Tan-Lim C.S.C. et al. (2021)	Different strains of *Bifidobacterium* and *Lactobacillus*	In a review study, the authors compared the effects of several probiotics on the AD course. The most effective were: • Complex№ 1 (*Bifidobacterium animalis subsp lactis, Bifidobacterium longum, Lactobacillus casei*) • *Lactobacillus casei* • Complex№ 6 (*Bifidobacterium bifidum, Lactobacillus acidophilus, Lactobacillus casei,* and *Lactobacillus salivarius*) Compared to placebo, Complex№ 1 reduced AD symptoms with a high degree of certainty, Complex№ 6 with a moderate degree of certainty, and *Lactobacillus casei* with a low degree of certainty.

4.4.2. Topical administration of probiotics

Unlike oral probiotic products, which contain live microorganisms, topical probiotics are the result of special processing (fermentation, ultrasound treatment, heat treatment, etc.) of live strains, during which active substances are extracted from the bacterial biomass (Puebla-Barragan S., Reid G., 2021). Thus, **topical probiotics are not whole microorganisms but extracts or cell fragments that positively affect skin immunity and the microbiome when applied to the skin**.

For example, a randomized, double-blind study involving AD patients compared the effects of emollients containing a topical probiotic of *Lactobacillus sakei* probio 65, isolated from the Korean product kimchi (fermented cabbage), with conventional emollients (Park S.B. et al., 2014). The probiotic emollients suppressed *S. aureus* colonization of the skin, strengthened the epidermal barrier, and contributed to the regression of AD symptoms.

Similarly, Myles I.A. et al.'s (2020) study of the effects of a topical probiotic containing *Roseomonas mucosa* demonstrated a marked reduction in disease severity, the need for topical steroids, and the degree of skin colonization by *Staphylococcus aureus* under the influence of the probiotic. The authors did not record any adverse events or complications. Most studies conducted to date have shown that probiotics have a positive effect on the AD course.

Table II-4-4 provides examples of skincare products containing topical probiotics.

Table II-4-4. Examples of skincare products containing topical probiotics (Gao T. et al., 2023)

PRODUCT	TOPICAL PROBIOTIC	EFFECTS
Okana	*Bacillus* fermentative extract	Helps to maintain skin firmness and elasticity, gives it smoothness.
Amperna Cream	Probiotic complex: *Lactobacillus acidophilus* *Lactobacillus rhamnosus*	Soothes irritated skin and relieves redness. Clinically tested for eczema, dermatitis, perioral dermatitis, rosacea, and acne-prone skin. Reduces the signs of photoaging.
Elissah Bio P2 Laviol Skin Care	16 types and 35 strains of bacteria including 14 *Bifidobacterium* and *Lactobacilli*	Strengthens the protective barrier against environmental aggressors and reduces susceptibility to factors that cause redness and irritation.
Melvory Probiotic Cream	*Lactobacillus* fermentative filtrate	Cleanses the skin of pathogenic bacteria. For acne-prone or teenage skin.
Andalou Naturals Probiotic+ C Renewal Cream	*Bacillus coagulans*	Probiotic microflora enzymatically supports dermal function for a brighter, tighter, more radiant complexion.
Biossance Squalane+ Probiotic Gel	*Lactococcus* enzymatic lysate	Promotes the restoration of the epidermal barrier.
Neogen Dermalogy Probiotics Double Action	Patented complex including enzymatic *Bifidobacterium* lysate, *Lactobacillus* lysate, and *Streptococcus thermophilus* enzymes	Improves skin barrier properties.

Continued on p. 131

PRODUCT	TOPICAL PROBIOTIC	EFFECTS
Elemis Dynamic Resurfacing Facial Pads	*Lactococcus* enzymatic lysate	Stimulates skin cell renewal, strengthens the epidermal barrier.
Manyo Factory Bifida Complex Ampoule	Enzymatic lysates of *Bifido-* and *Lactobacilli* as well as enzymatic lysate of *Lactococcus* spp.	Promotes regeneration and increases skin moisturization, prevention of age-related changes.
LaFlore Probiotic Serum Concentrate	*Lactococcus* enzymatic lysate and live kefir probiotics (*Hansenula / Kloeckera / Lactobacillus / Lactococcus / Leuconostoc / Pediococcus / Saccharomyces*)	Smoothens microrelief, reduces wrinkles, strengthens the skin's natural protective barrier.
Elizabeth Arden Superstart Probiotic Boost Skin Renewal Biocellulose Mask	*Lactococcus* enzymatic lysate, inactivated strains of *Lactobacillus casei* and *Lactobacillus acidophilus*	Optimizes the composition of the skin microbiome, strengthens the epidermal barrier, moisturizes and smoothens the skin.
Dot and Key 72 h Hydrating Gel and Probiotics	Fermented by *Saccharomyces* black tea extract, *Lactobacillus* spp.	Provides long-lasting moisturization, restores the microbiome balance.

Chapter 5
Skincare tools for preventing and treating signs of skin aging and aesthetic conditions in atopic patients

Atopic patients are characterized by the premature appearance of age-related skin changes. The main culprits behind this phenomenon are the apparent features of atopic skin — insufficient resistance to external destructive factors due to a broken epidermal barrier. However, hidden causes also act from within. Immune dysfunction, one of the main factors in the pathogenesis of AD, is the basis for persistent chronic inflammation, which, even in remission, can smolder asymptomatically and contribute to the skin aging process.

We will start by discussing the modern skincare approaches that can be adopted for treating atopic skin. By considering the role of chronic inflammation in aging, we will better understand the features of atopic skin and justify the choice of specific cosmetic products and procedures.

5.1. Inflammation and preventive anti-aging strategies

The term "inflammaging" is a portmanteau combining "inflammation" and "aging" as a reference to aging due to inflammation. This concept was first mentioned in the scientific press in 2000. In the *Annals of the New York Academy of Sciences*, it was proposed by Claudio Franceschi, a renowned Italian immunologist and professor at the University of Bologna (**Fig. II-5-1**). What is inflammation, and how can we influence it?

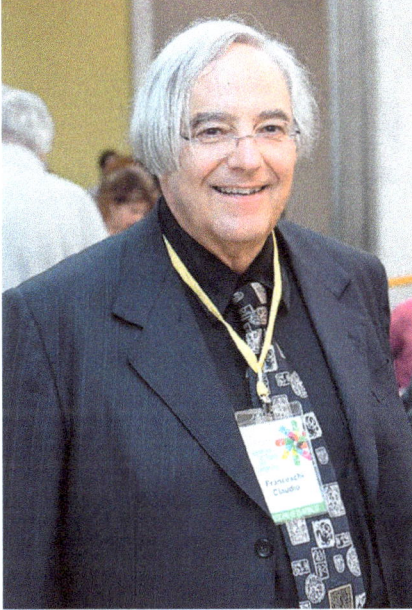

Figure II-5-1. Claudio Franceschi at the Genetics of Aging and Longevity Conference (April 22, 2012)

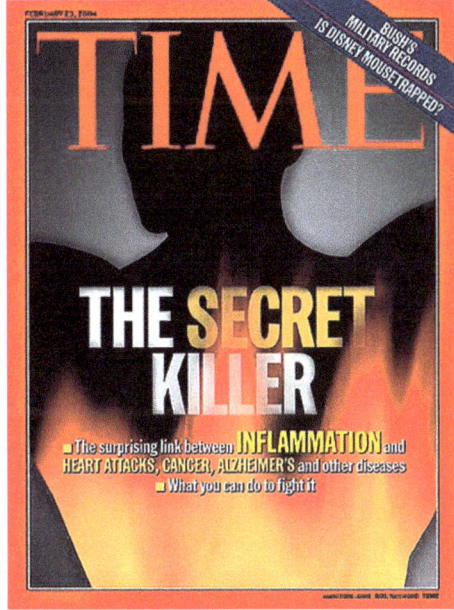

Figure II-5-2. Cover of the *Time* magazine (February 2004)

Franceschi's main idea is that chronic inflammation, which can be subtle, i.e., without vivid clinical symptoms or asymptomatic, undermines the body's vitality (including the skin) and accelerates the aging processes in all organs and systems.

In 2004, an intriguing headline, "The Secret Killer," appeared on the cover of *Time* magazine (**Fig. II-5-2**). In the article associated with this title, the authors discussed the link between inflammation and neoplasms, heart attacks, Alzheimer's disease, and many other ailments. They argued that internal inflammation can contribute to the emergence of various diseases, including those serious enough to be fatal.

Since the 2000s, physicians of various specialties have actively studied and discussed the topic, identifying the key features of inflammation.

1. **Asymptomatic course and insignificant severity:** a person does not notice inflammation
2. **Controllability:** when it is known that such inflammation is present in the body, it can be controlled or eliminated

3. **Non-pathologic in nature:** inflammation does not destroy tissues at the affected site
4. **Chronic course:** inflammation can last for years without any outward signs
5. **Presence of systemic inflammatory changes:** all are virtually invisible in daily life
6. **Positive effects on the body in the early stages of inflammation and adverse effects in the later stages of inflammation**

The immune system is the key player in inflammaging, leading to events that result in visible age-related changes.

This concept of inflammaging overlaps with one of the evolutionary theories of aging — antagonistic pleiotropy. In a nutshell, its essence is "delayed payback." What is beneficial for existence and survival at the beginning of our lives becomes detrimental at later stages and only accelerates aging by maintaining a "smoldering" inflammatory focus or multiple foci.

5.1.1. Causes of inflammaging and the competence of the skincare practitioner

Skin inflammation can develop against the background of chronic **somatic diseases** accompanied by inflammatory processes that, if untreated, eventually result in sluggish inflammation.

One of the causes of inflammation is **irrational nutrition** due to the overconsumption of high-calorie foods rich in carbohydrates and fats (Agrawal R. et al., 2023). This sets the stage for asymptomatic inflammation in the body, not only at the skin level (**Fig. II-5-3**).

Solar radiation also contributes to local inflammatory lesions in areas regularly exposed to the sun. These lesions can be visible but also hidden by a dark tan.

Regular **skin irritation**, such as allergies, mechanical friction, etc., can also lead to the emergence of a chronic inflammatory focus, which literally "undermines" the health of the skin and the entire body from within.

Frequent traumatic aesthetic procedures (usually chemical peeling) with breaks that are insufficient for full recovery can also lead to a state of prolonged sluggish inflammation that undermines skin health.

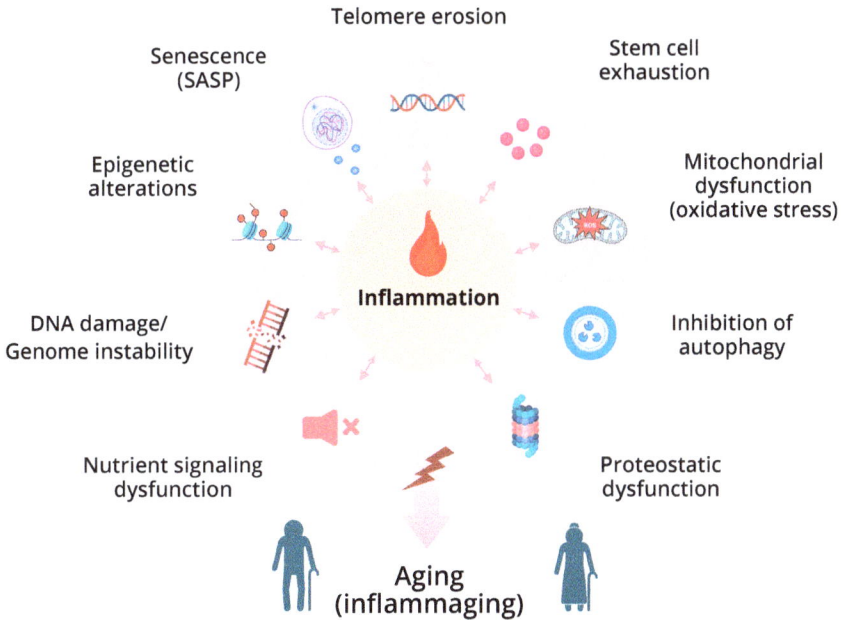

Figure II-5-3. Linking aging mechanisms and chronic inflammation (Agrawal R. et al., 2023)

The mechanisms thought to underlie the aging process include proteostatic dysfunction, inhibition of autophagy, mitochondrial dysfunction (which results in increased oxidative stress), stem cell exhaustion, telomere erosion, senescence (and the associated senescence-associated secretory program, or SASP), epigenetic alterations, DNA damage and genomic instability, and nutrient signaling dysfunction. These mechanisms often increase inflammation, which leads to inflammaging.

Which of these causes of inflammation can be addressed by an aesthetician?

Aestheticians can competently prescribe treatments with adequate recovery and appropriate "rest time." They can also recommend sufficient sun protection to reduce the amount of insolation on the skin. Finally, they can work with the skin manifestations of allergic reactions (to a certain extent), the effects of mechanical irritation, etc.

Although somatic pathologies and dietary recommendations are beyond the competence of estheticians, their expertise is sufficient to help many patients suffering from inflammation.

5.1.2. Factors contributing to inflammaging

Substances that set off inflammatory reactions in our body are called pro-inflammatory triggers. These include cytokines (IL-1, -4, -6, -10, -12, and -18, TNFα, INF-γ, TGF-β) and chemokines (IL-8, monocyte chemostatic factor 1 — MCP-1).

Under the influence of triggers, **inflammation markers** —hypoxia-inducible factor 1α (HIF-1α) and vascular endothelial growth factor (VEGF) — appear in the blood.

Inflammation also contributes to the development of inflammation:

- **Reactive oxygen species (ROS)** are chemical compounds in which oxygen has an unpaired electron in an outer orbital. Their levels vary with UV exposure and the presence of antioxidant enzymes (**Fig. II-5-4**). If excess ROS are not deactivated promptly, they damage lipids, proteins, and the cell genome through oxidation. UV radiation (especially its long-wavelength component — UVA) induces reactive oxygen species.
- **Tumor necrosis factor α (TNFα)** is a multifunctional pro-inflammatory cytokine synthesized mainly by monocytes and macrophages. It influences lipid metabolism, blood coagulation, and endothelial function. It also stimulates the production of IL-1, -6, -8, and INF-γ and activates leukocytes.
- **Interleukin-6** is a cytokine that can have both pro- and anti-inflammatory effects. Activated macrophages and T cells synthesize it.
- **Neutrophils** are granulocytic leukocytes that phagocytize relatively small foreign particles or cells. They subsequently usually die, releasing large amounts of biologically active substances that increase inflammation and activate the chemotaxis of immune cells into the nidus.
- **Matrix metalloproteinases (MMPs)** are a family of extracellular zinc-dependent endopeptidases capable of degrading all extracellular matrix proteins.
- The **complement system** is a complex of proteins constantly present in the blood. It is a cascade of proteolytic enzymes designed to defend the body against foreign agents and is involved in immune response.

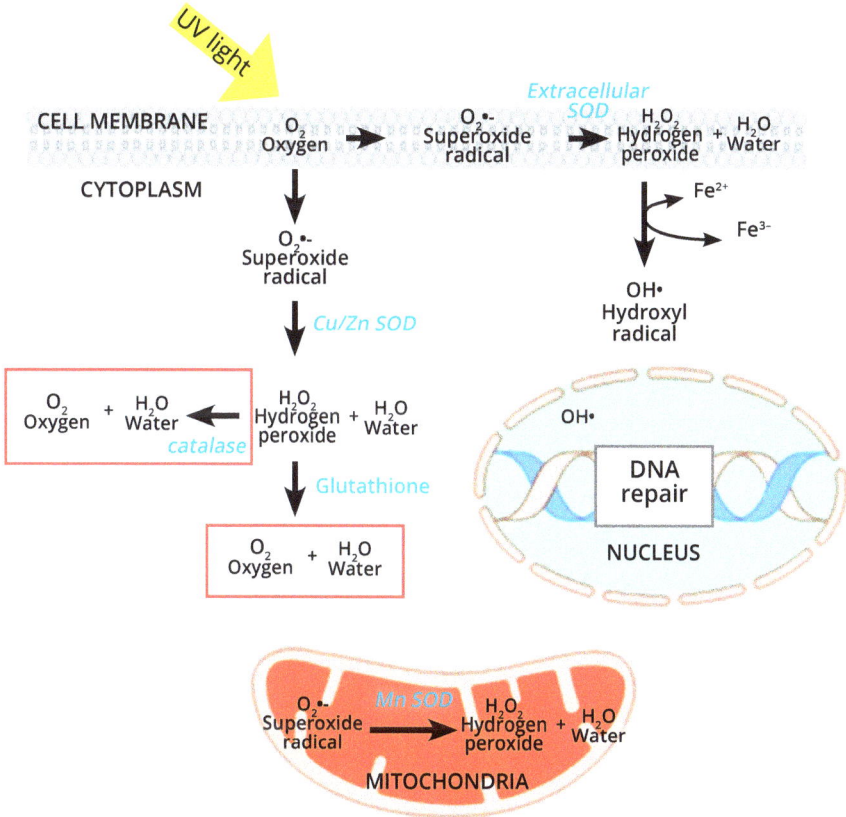

Figure II-5-4. Cellular antioxidant defenses (adapted from Amaro-Ortiz A. et al., 2014)

UV radiation induces the production of various ROS, which alter the molecular structure and damage lipids, proteins, and nucleic acids because of their chemical reactivity. Antioxidant enzymes mediate the removal of ROS, with different enzymes functioning in specific compartments (e.g., Mn SOD localized to mitochondria). ROS may react with DNA and other cell signal proteins, impairing their function if not removed. SOD — extracellular superoxide dismutase. Cu/Zn SOD — copper/zinc superoxide dismutase. Mn SOD — manganese superoxide dismutase.

■ **Macrophages** are cells capable of actively capturing and digesting bacteria, remnants of dead cells, and other particles foreign or toxic to the body. The number of macrophages of monocytic origin increases sharply during inflammation and normalizes after its termination.

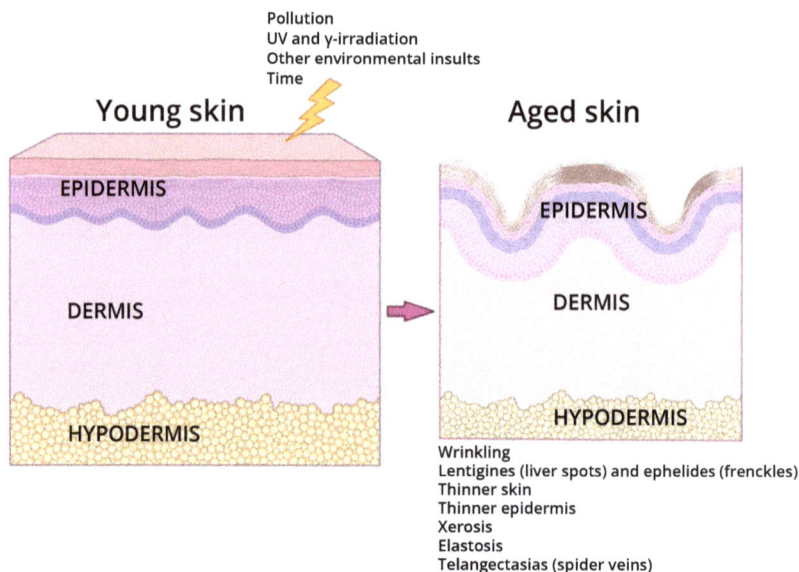

Young skin · Aged skin

Pollution
UV and γ-irradiation
Other environmental insults
Time

EPIDERMIS
DERMIS
HYPODERMIS

EPIDERMIS
DERMIS
HYPODERMIS

Wrinkling
Lentigines (liver spots) and ephelides (frenckles)
Thinner skin
Thinner epidermis
Xerosis
Elastosis
Telangectasias (spider veins)

Figure II-5-5. Aging skin. Over time, aging skin undergoes several changes, leading to its dysfunction. Some unfavorable external factors can accelerate natural aging (adapted from Agrawal R. et al., 2023)

5.1.3. Skin inflammaging hallmarks

In addition to the biochemical signs of inflammaging, there are clinical hallmarks.

The skin's **roughness** and **dullness** are most often caused by the slowdown of epidermal cell renewal (**Fig. II-5-5**). This process occurs against the background of certain histological phenomena: spongiosis (intercellular edema), tissue acidification (decrease in pH), and hypoxia, which inhibit keratinocyte proliferation and differentiation.

Skin laxity and **deep wrinkles** may also be noticeable in patients with inflammaging — they are symptoms of more profound structural changes, including those to the dermal matrix. The underlying pathogenetic mechanisms are similar to the appearance of dull skin — spongiosis, tissue acidification, and hypoxia, against the background of which MMPs are activated, and the synthetic activity of fibroblasts is reduced.

Pigment disorders such as dyschromia and age spots may occur against the background of hypoxia and tissue acidification, which modify melanogenesis and pigment distribution.

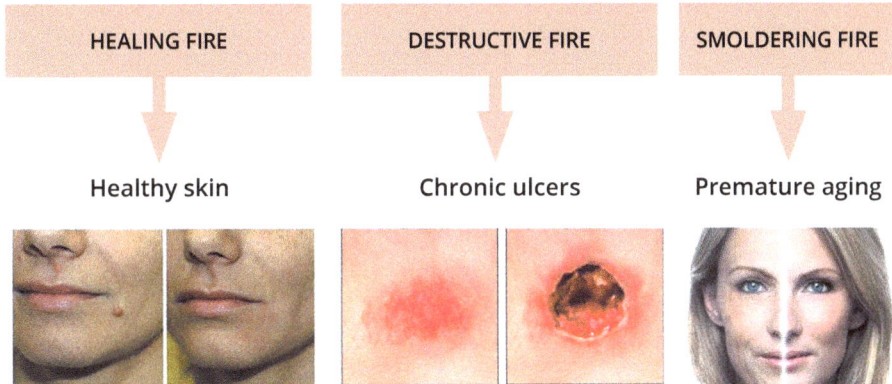

| HEALING FIRE | DESTRUCTIVE FIRE | SMOLDERING FIRE |

Healthy skin   Chronic ulcers   Premature aging

Figure II-5-6. Three types of inflammation

Lipoatrophy is also a clinical symptom of inflammation. Changes in the subcutaneous fatty tissue occur for the reasons mentioned above. An "inflammatory fire" that has not been extinguished in time causes the skin to age faster.

Inflammation can be "bad" as well as "good." Different types of inflammation can be compared to a healing fire, a destructive wildfire, or a smoldering bonfire. In the first case, inflammation promotes skin rejuvenation by eliminating or literally "burning out" the defect, after which healthy skin forms in its place. Inflammation benefits the skin and the entire body, resulting in a favorable outcome. A destructive wildfire is formed when uncontrolled inflammation leads to chronic ulcers and other defects. Finally, the smoldering bonfire of inflammation is something we don't notice in our daily lives, but it constantly, day after day, undermines our skin's resources, leading to premature aging — inflammaging (**Fig. II-5-6**).

5.1.4. Inflammaging monitoring

How do we identify hidden inflammation?

We have at least three objective tests at our disposal:
1. **Tewametry** for TEWL assessment
2. **Thermometry** for surface temperature assessment
3. **Mexametry** for erythema assessment

Tewametry records passive water transport through the *stratum corneum* to the external environment. When an inflammatory lesion occurs, the overlying skin gradually loses its barrier function, causing TEWL to increase.

Thermometry is also needed to look for localized inflammation because it is associated with a temperature increase.

Mexametry assesses the degree of erythema, which is very useful for tanned skin, where redness is challenging to see with the naked eye.

5.1.5. Anti-ageing care strategy for atopic skin

Continuous control of inflammation is a crucial part of anti-aging therapy and skincare. Its objectives are summarized below:
1. **Protection** against UV damage, excessive dryness, physical damage, etc. — sunscreens, emollients, moisturizers, etc.
2. **Inflammation management** — antioxidants, anti-inflammatory agents
3. **Itch reduction** — synthetic peptide Neurosensine™ (INCI: Acetyl Dipeptide-1 Cetyl Ester)
4. **Comprehensive post-treatment care to restore skin integrity** — physiological lipids (ceramides, cholesterol, free fatty acids), sebum-like substances (squalene, waxes, saturated fatty alcohols, etc.)

Sunscreens with a maximal sun protection factor (SPF) should not be used unless necessary. In the middle latitudes, SPF 10–20 is sufficient. Many day creams include a small amount of UV filters and thus provide adequate skin protection. To control inflammation, preparations containing antioxidants and anti-inflammatory agents can be used. Synthetic peptide Neurosensine™ can be applied to reduce itching, as it blocks neurogenic inflammation (i.e., its action is similar to strontium nitrate, which is rarely prescribed nowadays). By helping to eliminate the "consequences of destruction," we are effectively restoring the integrity of the skin.

The basic principles of anti-aging therapy as applied to inflammaging:
1. Use of anti-inflammatory agents to prevent and treat inflammation

2. Special preparation of the skin before traumatic procedures to strengthen its regenerative potential
3. Actively helping the damaged skin to repair to avoid acute in-flammation from becoming chronic
4. Competent prescription of aesthetic treatment accompanied by inflammation — without "abusing" the possibilities of cosmetic dermatology

5.2. Peculiarities of aesthetic correction of atopic skin

The skin of women with AD ages faster (**Fig. II-5-7**) than that of their healthy counterparts. Therefore, the need for anti-aging care arises earlier, but high skin sensitivity often leads these women to avoid beauty salons. Peculiarities of care for atopic skin:

- Combining basic care for atopic skin (see Part II, ch. 3) with anti-age care
- Hypersensitivity to the agents used
- Delayed repair
- The dependence of care on the stage of the disease

Cosmetic procedures can be performed in the long-term absence of exacerbations and relapses. Aesthetic treatments that weaken the *stratum corneum* should be avoided. Some cosmetic products and procedures can lead to barrier failure, such as:

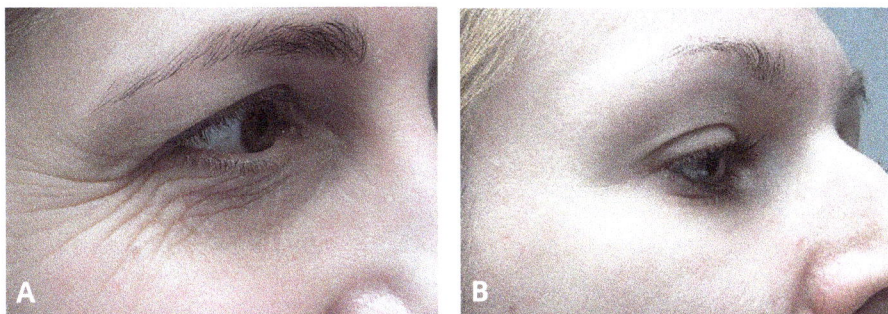

Figure II-5-7. Periorbital zone: A — a 38-year-old woman with AD, B — a 38-year-old healthy woman (photo provided by V.I. Albanova)

- Chemical peeling
- Retinol cosmetics
- Scrubs
- Microneedling
- Mechanical dermabrasion
- Laser dermabrasion
- Fractional ablative procedures such as radiofrequency (RF) microneedling, photothermolysis, plasma sublimation

Acute and chronic skin diseases also serve as general absolute contraindications for all types of hair removal.

As the above-mentioned means and methods damage the *stratum corneum*, they must be avoided or used with precautions. Let us examine the possibilities and limitations of aesthetic cosmetology methods in AD.

5.2.1. Chemical peeling

A chemical peel procedure involves the application of a chemical agent to the skin to cause controlled damage to the skin through chemical reactions between its structural elements and the chemical agent. The result is active exfoliation of the *stratum corneum* (**Fig. II-5-8**). Massive "shedding" of horny scales serves as a signal for basal keratinocytes to accelerate division to restore the skin barrier structures as soon as possible. Chemical peeling agents are preparations of intensive action that stimulate and accelerate the process of cell renewal in the epidermis (keratinocyte proliferation, migration, and differentiation) and the formation of barrier structures in the *stratum corneum* (keratinization and desquamation).

Any effect on the skin aimed at structural remodeling must rely on its ability to renew. The deeper the damage, the greater the strain on the skin's repair systems and the greater the chance that something in this repair process will go wrong. An inflammatory response can be an ally, but only if it is mild and disappears quickly. In contrast, the risk of complications increases if the inflammation is severe and chronic.

Midline and deep peels affect the epidermal living cells, so regeneration is needed. In atopic patients, genetically determined abnormalities

OUTSIDE-IN

Exfoliation through destruction or inhibition			**INSIDE-OUT** — Exfoliation through stimulation
Proteins' denaturation	Corneodesmosomes' hydrolysis	Changes in the activity of the *stratum corneum'* enzymes	Activation of basal keratinocyte proliferation and migration
• Phenol • TCA • Resorcinol • Salicylic acid • LHA	• Proteolytic enzymes	• AHAs • PHAs	• Retinol • Retinyl esters

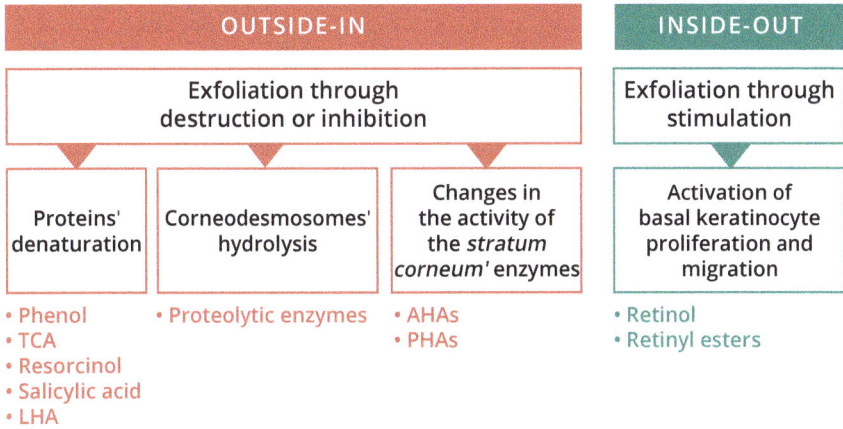

Figure II-5-8. "Outside-in" and "inside-out" peeling: principle of action and chemical agents

of the epidermal barrier and immune dysregulation impede the normal course of the regeneration process. The increased permeability of the *stratum corneum* facilitates the permeation of the applied chemical agent and enhances the immune system's response. This creates the basis for more pronounced inflammation and increases the risk of complications. For this reason, AD serves as a contraindication to midline and deep peels.

Practitioners should also consider the peel agents' mechanism of action, which depends on their chemical nature.

Atopic skin is characterized by thinning *stratum corneum*, increased surface pH values, altered activity of proteolytic enzymes, and sebum deficiency.

Given its peculiarities, let's consider a probable scenario of peel impact on atopic skin.

Keratolytic peeling

Keratolytic substances include phenol, trichloroacetic acid (TCA), salicylic acid, and resorcinol. Due to their high toxicity, phenol and TCA are currently banned from inclusion in cosmetic products.

Keratolytic agents break disulfide bonds that maintain proteins' three-dimensional configuration, denaturing all protein structures, including keratin, cornified envelope proteins, corneodesmosomes, proteolytic enzymes, and enzymes required for lipid barrier formation. This has a powerful destructive effect on the *stratum corneum*, which is already fragile and thinning in atopic patients, making such a pronounced keratolytic effect unwarranted and unnecessary.

Moreover, salicylic acid is a fat-soluble substance that quickly passes through the ducts of sebaceous glands, dissolves well in sebum, reaches sebocytes, and inhibits their synthetic activity. This leads to decreased sebum production and, consequently, reduced skin oiliness. However, as low sebum production is already a characteristic of AD, the influence of salicylic acid only aggravates the existing problem of sebum deficiency.

Therefore, **salicylic peeling should not be performed on patients with AD, even those in remission, to avoid exacerbating the disease**.

Enzymatic peeling

Enzymatic peels contain proteolytic enzymes of plant (bromelain, papain, ficin), microbiological (subtilisin), or synthetic (cross-papain) origin. Enzymatic peels are considered the mildest among chemical peels but have contraindications.

As mentioned earlier (see Part II, section 1.1.4), the surface pH of atopic skin is above the normal range. Against this background, the activity of protease inhibitors in the *stratum corneum* decreases, leading to an increase in protease activity that destroys the corneodesmosomes. As desquamation increases, the *stratum corneum* thins even more, weakening the epidermal barrier.

Enzymes are also proteins, and proteins are potential allergens. Given that immune dysfunction is involved in AD pathogenesis, the risks of an allergic reaction to a foreign protein are higher in AD patients than in healthy individuals.

Therefore, applying **enzymatic peels containing proteolytic enzymes that destroy the corneodesmosomes and enhance exfoliation is inappropriate.**

Retinol peeling

Retinol peeling —"inside-out" peeling — relies on retinol, the alcoholic form of vitamin A, as an active ingredient. Retinol is a fat-soluble substance that quickly passes through the *stratum corneum* without directly damaging enzymes or other components. Its main targets are basal keratinocytes and sebocytes. By acting on the genetic apparatus of living cells through specific nuclear receptors, retinol regulates the activity of many genes of all types of skin cells, including:

1. Keratinocyte genes that control cell division, maturation, and migration
2. Sebocyte genes responsible for sebum production

Thus, retinol accelerates the epidermal cell renewal processes and suppresses sebum production.

Retinol peels aggravate the low-sebum condition in atopic skin, cause the lipid barrier disorder, and increase TEWL. For this reason, this type of chemical peel is not recommended for individuals suffering from AD.

Acid peeling

Alpha-hydroxy acids (AHAs) are not keratolytic because they do not break covalent bonds within or between protein molecules and do not damage proteins. Their effect on skin physiology is to change the pH of the aqueous environment (acidification), which in turn affects ionic interactions between organic molecules and enzymatic activity in the *stratum corneum*.

The following biological effects are observed at the cellular and tissue level:

- Increase in mitotic activity of basal keratinocytes
- Increase in the number of lamellar bodies in granular keratinocytes
- Acceleration of cellular renewal in the epidermis
- Thinning of the *stratum corneum*
- Strengthening of the barrier function

The clinical impact of superficial acid peels will be a slight exfoliation of the *stratum corneum*, smoothing of the microrelief, and brightening of the skin tone. The following formulations can be used for atopic skin:

- 20–30% AHA, pH 2–3 — for superficial peel treatment in the office
- 5–10% AHA, pH 4–5 — for pre-peeling preparation at home

The best AHA for atopic skin is lactic acid, an NMF component. When applied to the skin, lactic acid is absorbed by the *stratum corneum*. Since it is hygroscopic, it binds water, increasing the *stratum corneum* hydration. This moisturizing effect lasts until the lactic acid is exfoliated along with the corneocytes to which it is bound. Typically, lactic acid is introduced into the treatment program at week 4 to exfoliate superficial skin layers and treat hyperkeratosis without compromising the barrier function. The interaction of lactic acid with ceramides and its ability to bind water makes it an essential component of dry, low-sebum skin therapy.

Lactic acid slightly inhibits tyrosinase, which makes it well-suited for depigmentation therapy. Its use for four weeks has a double effect:

1. Positive impact on the psychological state of the patient because, even after one treatment, the skin becomes cleaner and lighter
2. Tyrosinase inhibition slows down melanogenesis and promotes the efficacy of other depigmenting products

After a surface peeling, emollients containing an equimolar mixture of ceramides, cholesterol, and free fatty acids at a 1:1:1 ratio can be applied for faster recovery.

In sum, superficial acid peeling is the only viable option that still allows gentle smoothing of atopic skin while cleansing it from accumulated conglomerates of horny masses, sebum, and impurities. Although the effect of AHA is gentle, given the hypersensitivity of atopic skin, it is necessary to test the peel product by applying a small amount to the elbow area before carrying out the procedure.

For more information about chemical peeling, see our *Chemical Peeling in Cosmetic Dermatology & Skincare Practice* book.

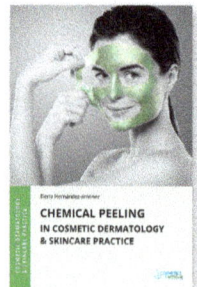

CHEMICAL PEELING
IN COSMETIC DERMATOLOGY
& SKINCARE PRACTICE

5.2.2. Aesthetic injections

Any dermatosis in acute form is a contraindication for injection procedures. However, adult patients with a favorable AD course may still be suitable candidates.

Can injectables be used during a period of relative clinical well-being? Two factors must be considered to answer this question.

First, you need to assess how traumatic the procedure itself is. It is one thing to have a few punctures to inject filler or botulinum toxin. It's quite another to have multiple, closely spaced punctures for mesotherapy — such severe trauma can trigger an disease exacerbation.

Second, you should remember the permanent dysfunction of the immune system in atopic patients. Even though AD in the long-term absence of exacerbations is not among the contraindications for injectable aesthetic treatment, the following recommendations should be heeded to prevent an allergic reaction:

- Taking an allergy history before the procedure
- Performing an allergy skin test
- Equipping the workplace with an allergy emergency kit

Below, we consider several of the most feasible drugs for injectable administration in terms of safety and efficacy.

Hyaluronic acid (HA) injections

Hyaluronic acid ($(C_{14}H_{21}NO_{11})n$) is the most common injectable material in aesthetic medicine. HA is a natural polysaccharide polymer found in the human intraocular media, synovial and pleural fluids, blood and lymph, and skin. The HA present in the dermis has systemic and regulatory functions, including being a water-holding matrix (**Fig. II-5-9**). HA is found in most multicellular and unicellular organisms (including many bacteria). It lacks species specificity, which makes it possible to use HA of any origin for medical purposes if adequately purified.

Different forms of HA are used in aesthetic injections:
1. Modified (cross-linked) HA for volume restoration (face and body contouring with dermal HA fillers)
2. Non-modified (native) HA for skin restructuration (mesotherapy)

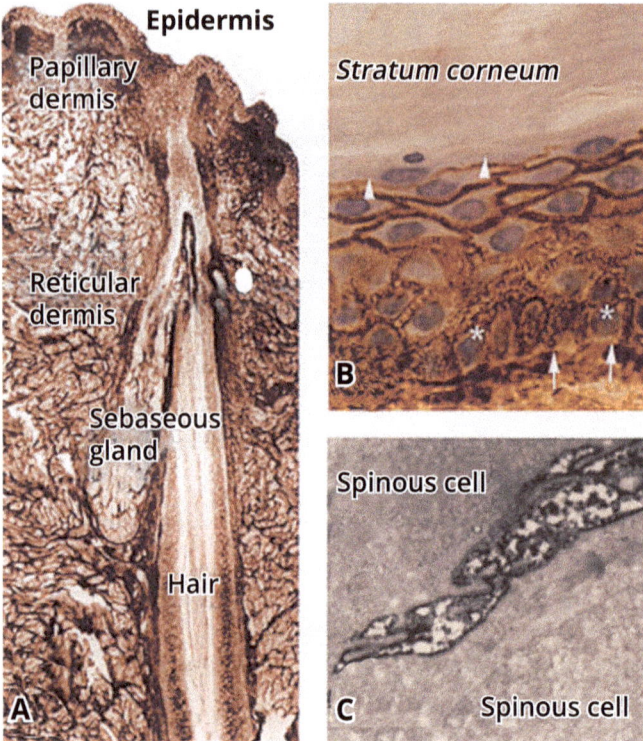

Figure II-5-9. Hyaluronan in adult human skin (adapted from Tammi R. et al., 1988)

Human skin sections were stained for hyaluronan using biotinylated G1 protein and link protein complex. The binding of the complex was visualized using the avidin-biotin-peroxidase technique (in a, brown), and nuclei were counterstained with hematoxylin (in b, blue). Intense staining is present in the epidermis from the basal layer (asterisk) up to the granular cell layer (arrowheads). The connective tissue below the basal lamina (papillary dermis) is strongly positive, whereas the deeper connective tissue (reticular dermis) shows moderate staining intensity. Epithelial cells in the skin appendages (sebaceous glands and hair follicles) are also stained. Arrows in (b) indicate the basal lamina. (c) Ultrastructural localization of hyaluronan in human epidermis. Human skin sections were stained for hyaluronan as described and then processed for transmission electron microscopy. The dark precipitate in the extracellular pouches between the keratinocytes indicates hyaluronan.

HA fillers are characterized by high biocompatibility and the absence of immune reactions, so they are the best choice for atopic patients. However, it should be remembered that, in atopic skin, HA degrades faster. In the focus of inflammation, tissues are under oxidative stress, and oxidative reactions accelerate the biodegradation of hyaluronic polymers. Therefore, before HA filler injection, an atopic patient should be warned that the volumetric effect may be less pronounced than in people without AD.

As for mesotherapy, the main limitation here will be the reaction of atopic skin to multiple skin micro-traumas caused by the needle. Thus, it is better not to take risks and avoid such interventions.

PRP therapy

Platelets play a central role in the healing and regeneration of damaged tissues by releasing growth factors that regulate and stimulate cell division, growth, and survival. Growth factors guide the reconstruction of blood vessels, the building of new tissue (epithelial, cartilage, connective, muscle, nerve), and stopping bleeding in the injured area (Solakoglu Ö. et al., 2020).

Platelet-rich plasma (PRP) is an autologous serum containing high concentrations of platelets and growth factors. Normal blood platelet concentration varies between 150,000/µl and 350,000/µl and averages at 200,000/µl, and PRP contains about 1,000,000/µl platelets. It also contains platelet-derived growth factors (PDGF-aa, PDGF-bb, PDGF-ab), transforming growth factors (TGF-β1, TGF-β2), vascular endothelial growth factor (VEGF), and epithelial growth factor (EGF). These natural growth factors are in biologically predetermined ratios. All this distinguishes PRP from preparations containing recombinant growth factors.

PRP intradermal injections (PRP therapy) are used to treat age-related changes and hallmarks of photodamage and promote healing (Emer J., 2019). They are an essential treatment modality with many applications in dermatology, particularly in skin rejuvenation, acne scars, *striae distensae*, and hair restoration.

Since PRP is derived from the patient's blood, it does not pose a risk of infection spread or adverse immune response. It is also free from potentially dangerous pathogens (foreign chemicals and microbes) and carries no risks of rejection, allergic reactions, or other adverse events. Therefore, it is particularly popular for atopic patients. At the same time, it is worth remembering the extensive trauma caused by the needle and being particularly attentive to the reaction of atopic skin to mechanical damage.

There is growing evidence on the efficacy of PRP therapy in treating AD, which can shorten the interval between refractory relapses (i.e., not responsive to conventional systemic treatment) and improve overall patient satisfaction due to its anti-inflammatory and regenerative properties. PRP not only suppresses the expression of inflammatory genes but also promotes tissue repair by creating a favorable environment for healing. It restores communication among keratinocytes, fibroblasts, and melanocytes and attracts and stimulates undifferentiated stem cells. The use of PRP therapy in the treatment of AD has been recognized as safe, including during pregnancy (Zaki S.N. et al., 2024).

Botulinum therapy

The two main aesthetic applications for botulinum therapy are expression line treatment and facial harmonization. During the procedure, botulinum toxin is injected deep under the skin — into the target muscle. It can be delivered through just one or a few injections, so mechanical trauma to the skin is minimal. Atopic dermatitis is not a contraindication for this procedure, so it can be used as a therapeutic tool to improve the skin condition of atopic patients.

Botulinum toxin type A (BTA) has demonstrated its therapeutic properties in treating rosacea, acne, and alopecia and is also used to lessen post-surgical scarring. Recently, atopic dermatitis was added to the list of potential indications for using BTA, which opens new horizons in treating this congenital dermatosis.

Khattab F.M. (2020) conducted a pilot study to evaluate the efficacy of BTA in treating atopic dermatitis. The experimental design included 20 patients with chronic moderate AD. BTA was administered as intradermal injections into the affected skin areas. The dosage was two units per point, with an injection interval of 1–2 cm. The total volume of toxin injected varied depending on the lesion location. Patients showed significant improvement in their clinical skin condition four weeks after treatment as measured by the SCORAD index. Itching — one of the most distressing symptoms of atopic dermatitis — was reduced by more than 50% in 80% of the study participants. In addition, patients noticed a reduction in skin redness and thickening.

BTA's effectiveness in treating atopic dermatitis is explained by its effect on nociceptors — the nerve endings responsible for the perception of pain and itching. BTA blocks the release of acetylcholine from presynaptic endings, reducing the activation of sensitive nerve fibers. Botulinum toxin is also thought to inhibit the release of neuropeptides such as SP and CGRP, which play a key role in inflammation and itching (Gazerani P., 2018; Gharib K. et al., 2020).

When administered intradermally, BTA acts on nerve endings and skin cells, including keratinocytes, fibroblasts, and immune cells. It suppresses the activation of keratinocytes, which are involved in inflammatory reactions, and reduces the secretion of pro-inflammatory cytokines. The effect on fibroblasts improves skin regeneration, and modulation of immune cell activity minimizes the severity of inflammation (Heckmann M. et al., 2002). This versatile action yields the following clinical effects:

1. Reduction in the itching intensity
2. Reduction in skin redness and swelling
3. Improvement of the barrier function of the epidermis
4. Reduced inflammation
5. Overall improvement in the quality of life of AD patients

Despite impressive results, using BTA in AD treatment is presently in the initial stages. More extensive clinical trials involving more patients are needed to confirm the efficacy and safety of this therapy mode. Nevertheless, botulinum toxin already shows excellent potential, opening new opportunities for treating chronic skin diseases.

Carboxytherapy

Carboxytherapy is a non-surgical treatment to improve the appearance of cellulite, stretch marks, and dark under-eye circles. It is performed by injecting carbon dioxide (CO_2) — a natural vasodilator — beneath the skin through a fine needle or by applying a CO_2-saturated gel onto the skin. In response to the CO_2 intake, blood vessels dilate, and local blood flow increases, activating metabolic processes. In addition, CO_2 promotes new vessel formation and improves microcirculation due to the VGF activation. Under the influence of CO_2, adipocytes are destroyed, and the released triglycerides enter the intercellular space.

In aesthetic medicine, carboxytherapy is used to treat the following conditions:

- Skin atony and low elasticity
- Wrinkles
- Age-related skin changes
- Fat deposits
- Gynoid lipodystrophy (cellulite)
- Stretchmarks
- Scars (incl. keloids)

Based on biological laws, carboxytherapy is a gentle intervention in physiological processes. It is essential in AD, which is characterized by a compromised epidermal barrier and immune dysregulation.

Atopic patients can use topical carboxytherapy without concern; injectable carboxytherapy must be performed cautiously due to the inevitable mechanical damage by the needle.

5.2.3. Energy-based treatments

Given the weakening of the epidermal barrier, thinning of the *stratum corneum*, dryness, and hypersensitivity of atopic patients, physical factors and technologies that significantly impact the superficial layer of the skin should be avoided, especially on the face and neck. However, several physical modalities focus on a deeper level, minimizing the effects on the fragile superficial skin layers. From this point of view, the following procedures are possible in atopic patients:

- **Photorejuvenation (by IPL)** can be performed at low energy levels, and it is advisable to use red/near-infrared light for anti-inflammatory impact.
- Despite its destructive effect, **laser treatment for age spots and vascular abnormalities** can be performed on a small area.
- **High-intensity focused ultrasound (HIFU)** is used for face lifting and ptosis treatment. Ultrasound waves of 10.0/7.0/4.0 MHz with a depth of focus of 1.5/3.0/4.5 mm affect the superficial muscle-aponeurotic system (SMAS) layer without violating the integrity of overlying tissues.

- **High-intensity focused electromagnetic energy (HIFEM)** for body contouring targets muscle and fat tissues.
- **Non-ablative RF** warms the dermal layer without damaging the epidermis, thickening the skin and smoothing wrinkles.
- **Photoepilation** removes unwanted hair.

Not recommended:

- **Cryolipolysis** — although the epidermis remains intact, ischemia occurs against the prolonged cooling of adipose tissue, and local blood circulation is impaired, which can trigger AD exacerbation.
- **Fractional interventions (laser- or RF-assisted microneedling)** cause extensive damage and are not recommended even in remission. Nevertheless, there is a report in the medical press about the successful use of fractional CO_2 laser for treating amyloid lichen on the body of an atopic patient (Chu H. et al., 2017), as well as the use of erbium-doped yttrium-scandium-gallium-garnet (Er:YSGG) laser for treating pigmented circles under the eyes (Park K.Y. et al., 2013).

For more information about physical modalities, see our *Lasers in Cosmetic Dermatology and Skincare Practice* and *Microcurrent, Ultrasound, and LED Therapy in Cosmetic Dermatology & Skincare Practice* books.

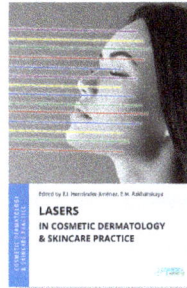

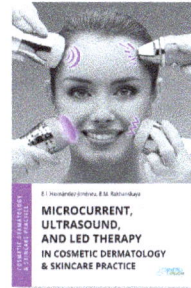

Atopic patient at the aesthetician's office

An atopic patient requires special attention. Many modern technologies and cosmetic products do not have AD on the list of contraindications. Still, the risk of adverse events remains higher because hypersensitivity and a weakened skin barrier can turn the skin response to a physical or chemical influence in an unpredictable direction. Therefore, it is up to the skincare practitioner and the patient to weigh the pros and cons of different treatment modalities. Taking informed consent, whereby the patient explicitly confirms their awareness of the risks associated with the procedure and documents this consent and willingness to bear responsibility for possible adverse health effects, can protect the specialist while prompting the potential client to consider the need for a particular intervention.

Refusing to explore the expansive possibilities of cosmetic dermatology or, conversely, ignoring the existing disease and resorting to any aesthetic treatment are two extremes. Between them, there is still a golden mean, requiring professionalism, deep knowledge from the specialist, and a reasonable attitude toward health from the patient.

Part III

Psoriasis

Chapter 1
Psoriasis as a chronic inflammatory disease

Psoriasis is among the most common and well-studied immune-mediated chronic skin diseases, affecting about 2–3% of the population worldwide, representing over 125 million patients (Chovatiya R., Silverberg J.I., 2019).

Thus, aestheticians are bound to encounter this condition in their practice. Understanding the pathogenesis of the disease is necessary for choosing appropriate aesthetic intervention strategies and providing effective counseling on basic skincare.

1.1. Understanding the pathogenesis of psoriasis. Are keratinocytes or immune cells the main culprit?

Chronic inflammation is the hallmark of psoriasis, leading to uncontrolled keratinocyte proliferation and impaired differentiation (**Fig. III-1-1**).

Early epidemiologic studies led scientists to believe that there is a genetic predisposition to psoriasis, as patients with psoriasis have a higher incidence of this condition among first- and second-degree relatives compared to the general population, and monozygotic twins have a 2–3 times higher risk of psoriasis than dizygotic twins (Chovatiya R., Silverberg J.I., 2019).

The classic cutaneous presentation of psoriasis is scaly erythematous plaques, localized or widely distributed. Up to 30% of patients with psoriasis could develop psoriatic arthritis. Moderate-to-severe psoriasis is associated with an increased risk of metabolic syndrome and cardiovascular disease (Yan B.X. et al., 2021).

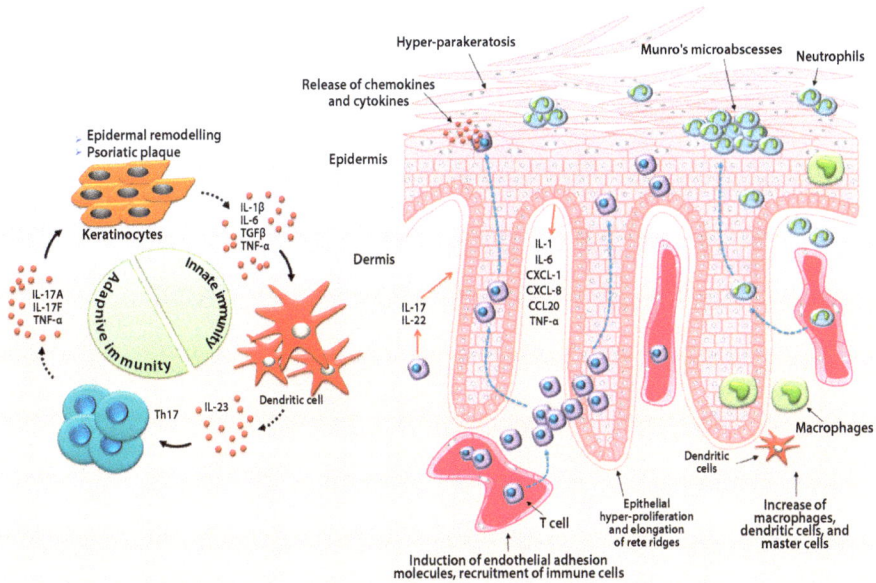

Figure III-1-1. Pathogenetic mechanisms of psoriasis nidus formation (adapted from Huang T.H. et al., 2019)

About 70 chromosome loci participating in the psoriasis manifestation (psoriasis susceptibility loci — PSORS) have been identified. They are located on different chromosomes, e.g., PSORS1 on 6p21.3, PSORS2 on 17q, PSORS3 on 4q, PSORS4 on 1q21, PSORS5 on 3q21, PSORS6 on 19p, PSORS7 on 1p, PSORS8 on 16q, PSORS9 on 4q31, PSORS10 on 18p11, PSORS11 on 5q31–q33, PSORS12 on 20q13, etc. However, specific genes and their role in the development of different psoriasis types are still unclear (Grän F. et al., 2020).

Traditionally, psoriasis has been viewed as a systemic inflammatory autoimmune disease controlled by T cells. Genetically determined abnormalities of innate and acquired immune responses at the skin level and the epidermal barrier were considered to lead to the emergence and maintenance of inflammation in psoriasis lesions in response to unfavorable external factors.

It is believed that psoriatic plaques arise against the background of an inflammatory reaction in the epidermis. It is assumed that cells of the innate (dendritic cells — DC, macrophages, neutrophils) and

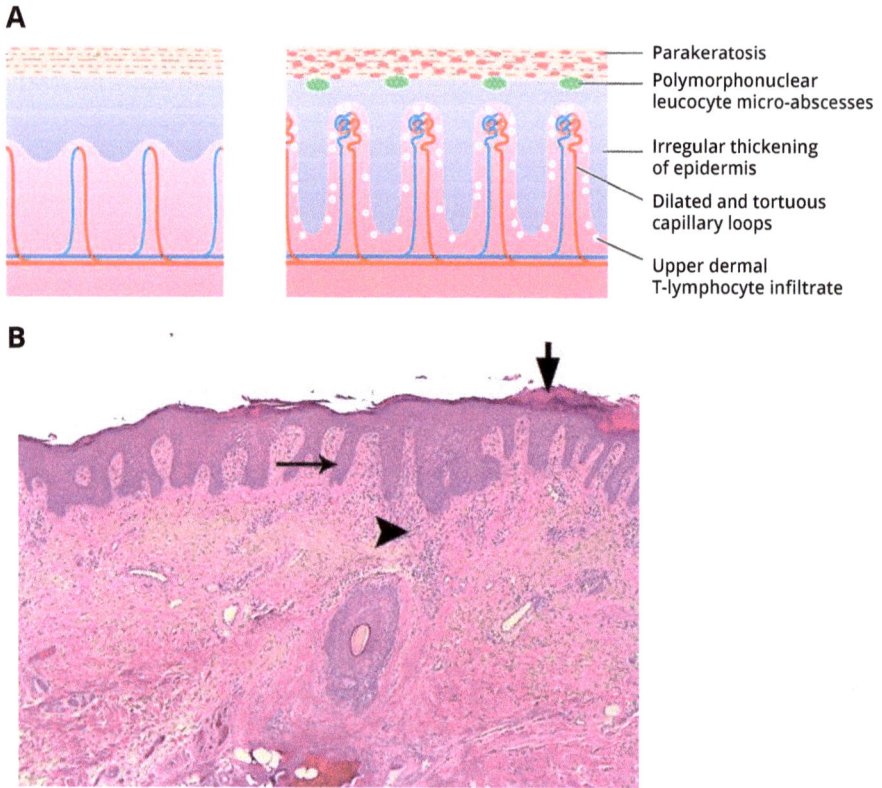

A

Parakeratosis

Polymorphonuclear leucocyte micro-abscesses

Irregular thickening of epidermis

Dilated and tortuous capillary loops

Upper dermal T-lymphocyte infiltrate

B

Figure III-1-2. Structural features of the skin in the psoriasis lesion

A — schematic representation; B — significant histologic changes in psoriasis skin: thickening of the epidermis (acanthosis) with regular elongation of epidermal ridges (long arrow), chronic inflammatory infiltrate in the upper layers of the dermis consisting mainly of small T cells (pointer arrow), and hyperkeratosis with parakeratosis (upper arrow)

acquired (B and T cells) immune system, as well as skin resident cells (keratinocytes, melanocytes), take part in such a response.

Histologic studies show specific alterations in the psoriasis skin lesions (**Fig. III-1-2**):

- A pronounced increase in the number of spiny epidermal cells (acanthosis)
- Thickening of the *stratum corneum* (hyperkeratosis)
- Disorder of epidermal cell keratinization, characterized by the presence of cells containing nuclei in the *stratum corneum* (parakeratosis)

- Massive infiltration of the skin with lymphocytes, macrophages, and neutrophils
- Increased density of skin capillaries with increased permeability in wide-caliber vessels

Yet, despite significant recent breakthroughs in understanding the pathophysiology of psoriasis, the order of these changes is not fully understood.

There are two main phases in the disease development:

1. The initiation phase of the inflammatory response
2. The self-sustaining phase of the chronic inflammation

The formation of the classic element in psoriasis — a scaly erythematous plaque — begins with the immune system stimulation by external triggers such as trauma, infection, and drugs. As a result of destructive factors, skin cells are damaged and begin to be perceived by the immune system as foreign (self-tolerance* disorder) — an inflammatory response occurs to fight against the epidermal cells. Let's take a closer look at how this happens.

In response to a trigger, keratinocytes secrete antimicrobial peptides (AMPs). The levels of these peptides are significantly higher in the skin of people with psoriasis. AMPs bind to the DNA of damaged cells, and the AMP–DNA complex can be perceived as foreign by immune cells. Dendritic cells (DCs) signal to T cells the presence of a "foreign agent" in the body through the production of interferon-alpha (IFN-α). T cells, in turn, secrete pro-inflammatory cytokines (TNFα, IL-6, -12, -17, -22, -23) in large quantities (Grän F. et al., 2020). Thus, the immune system begins to "fight" with keratinocytes.

IL-22 and IL-23 link the activation of immune cells and the functioning of keratinocytes. These pro-inflammatory mediators induce the proliferation of keratinocytes and their secretion of AMP and cytokines, which attract immune cells to the lesion. The circle is closed.

---

* Self-tolerance is the ability of the immune system to recognize self-produced antigens as a non-threat while appropriately mounting a response to foreign substances. Correctly balancing immunological defense and self-tolerance is critical to normal physiological function and overall health.

This pathological circle needs to be broken, and in this, along with drug therapy, skincare can help.

1.2. Disruption of the skin barrier function

According to statistics, 80% of patients trust exclusively local remedies, and with mild and moderate severity of psoriasis, local therapy is given absolute preference (Hashim P.W. et al., 2017). Understanding the skin's features in psoriasis is necessary to choose topical medicine, aesthetic treatment, and skincare products.

1.2.1. Biochemical markers of impaired epidermal barrier in psoriasis

Deletions in genes involved in the formation of the cornified envelope and keratinocyte differentiation cause primary defects of the epidermal barrier. Such disorders may underlie the abnormal reaction to external stimuli in psoriasis. Due to improper keratinocyte differentiation, the *stratum corneum* thickens but does not fulfill its protective function.

In psoriasis, the levels of prosaposin (involved in lipid metabolism), ceramides, and sphingomyelin — all cell membrane components — also decrease, indicating a disruption of the lipid barrier.

In addition to primary defects in the epidermal barrier, secondary disorders occur under chronic inflammation conditions: the inflammatory response interferes with the synthesis of structural components of the epidermal barrier, including filaggrin (Schmuth M. et al., 2015).

1.2.2. Dry skin and TEWL increase

According to extant studies, the TEWL rate is more than three times higher in psoriasis lesions than in healthy skin — 16.8 vs. 5.3 g/h/m^2. A significant difference is also observed when measuring the *stratum corneum* hydration: 4.7 units for psoriatic lesions vs. 42.4 units for healthy skin (Darlenski R. et al., 2018).

1.2.3. Hyperkeratosis and desquamation

It is believed that complete renewal of the epidermal cellular composition of the normal epidermis occurs in an average of 28–30 days. High levels of pro-inflammatory cytokines in psoriatic lesions stimulate keratinocyte proliferation, and epidermal renewal can be reduced to 5 days (Benhadou F. et al., 2019).

1.2.4. Hypersensitivity

Disruption of the epidermal barrier increases skin permeability to external factors, such as infection, chemicals, and solar radiation. Genetically determined loss of immune tolerance to foreign antigens and structural components of own tissues aggravates the situation, leading to increased immune system reactivity.

1.3. Microbiome alterations

1.3.1. Gut microbiome

The link between the gut microbiome and the immune system opens a new perspective for understanding the pathogenesis of many chronic inflammatory dermatoses, including psoriasis (Buhaş M.C. et al., 2022). The diversity of the gut microbiome may have a significant impact on the maturation of the immune system and the development of autoimmune diseases (Kierasińska M., Donskow-Łysoniewska K., 2021).

People with psoriasis show lower diversity and species composition changes in the gut microbiome compared to healthy individuals (Todberg T. et al., 2022). Metabolites produced by the gut microbiome have immunomodulatory potential to alter the balance between immune tolerance and inflammation by influencing the differentiation of naïve T cells into regulatory or Th17 lineages.

In patients with psoriasis, the microbiome is characterized by a decrease in the number of *Bacteroides* and *Proteobacteria* strains

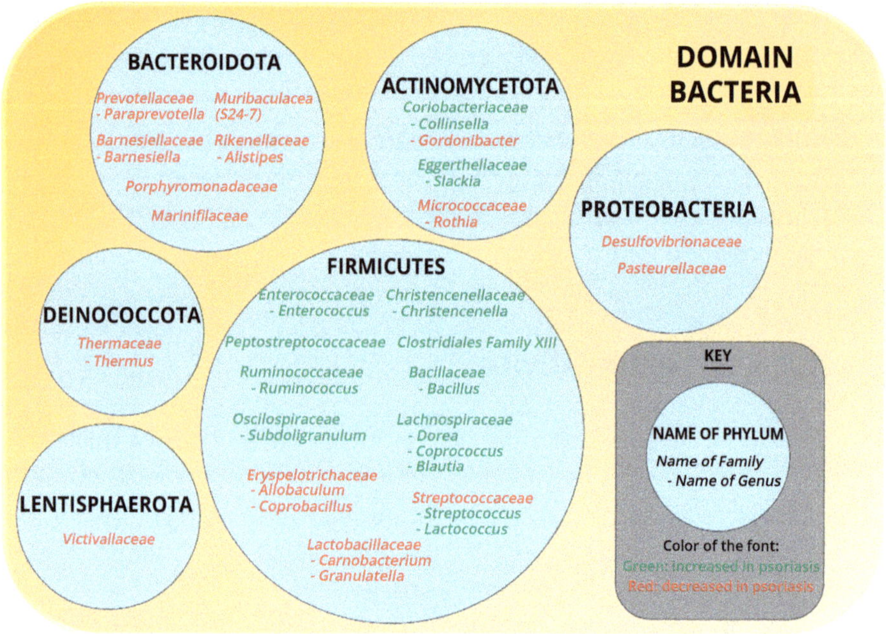

Figure III-1-3. Characteristic changes in the microbiome in psoriasis: population increase (green) and decrease (red) (adapted from Thye A.Y. et al., 2022)

and an increase in the proportion of *Actinobacteria* and *Firmicutes* (**Fig. III-1-3**) (Thye A.Y. et al., 2022). *Bacteroides* play an immunomodulatory role in the gut by producing polysaccharide A, which activates regulatory T cells (Visser M.J.E. et al., 2019).

A high proportion of *Firmicutes* has been shown in several studies to affect carbohydrate metabolism. These bacteria increase the production of acetates while decreasing the production of short-chain fatty acids (SCFAs) (**Fig. III-1-4**). At the same time, people with psoriasis are characterized by a decrease in an essential source of SCFAs, *F. prausnitzii*. This strain provides many benefits to the host organism as it is involved in the formation of butyrate (one of the short-chain fatty acids that give energy to colonocytes), reduces oxidative stress, and has anti-inflammatory effects by activating regulatory T cells, thus supporting immune tolerance that extends beyond the gastrointestinal tract (Eppinga H. et al., 2014). Decreased SCFA production can cause inflammation and weaken the intestinal epithelial barrier. Its integrity

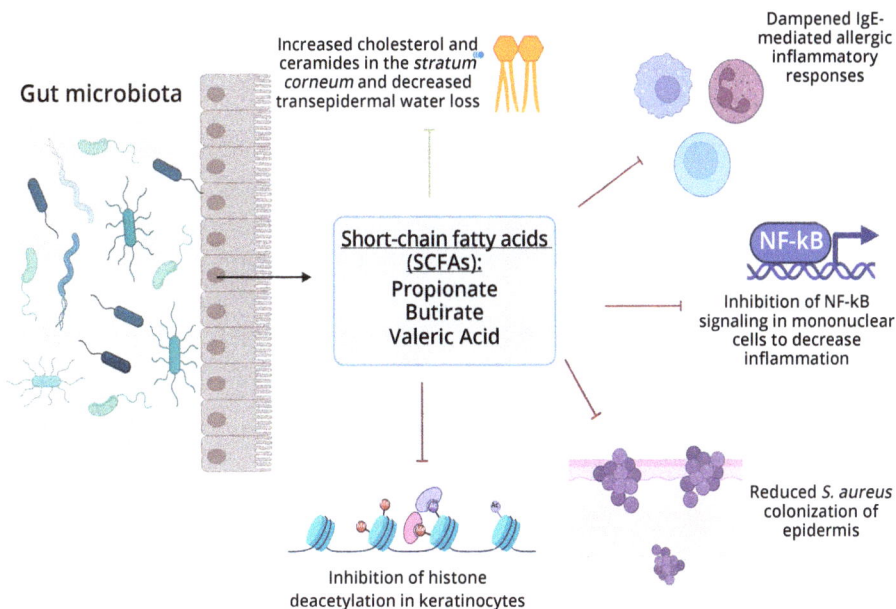

Figure III-1-4. Role of short-chain fatty acids in cutaneous immunity and epidermal homeostasis (adapted from Jiminez V., Yusuf N., 2023)

directly affects the process of antigen presentation and is responsible for maintaining immune balance. Weakening of the intestinal epithelial barrier affects both local and systemic immune responses.

Psoriasis is usually accompanied by inflammation in other organs, given that 7–11% of patients with inflammatory bowel disease (IBD) are diagnosed with psoriasis. Moreover, certain genetic and environmental factors and immune pathways are involved in the etiopathogenesis of both diseases. For example, Th17 cells and their cytokines, which are known to play a significant role in psoriasis, are also involved in the pathophysiology of IBD. This subset of cells is thought to be involved in developing ankylosing spondylitis and rheumatoid arthritis, two autoimmune inflammatory joint diseases commonly found in patients with psoriasis and IBD (Salem I. et al., 2018).

The pattern of dysbiosis in IBD has also been described in patients with psoriasis. There is a depletion of symbiont bacteria, including *Bifidobacteria*, *Lactobacilli*, and *Faecalibacterium prausnitzii*, as well as colonization by certain pathogenic microorganisms such as *Salmonella*, *Escherichia coli*, *Helicobacter*, *Campylobacter*, *Mycobacterium*, and *Alcaligenes*. Several studies show decreased *Parabacteroides* and *Coprobacillus* (two beneficial gut microbial species) counts in patients with psoriasis, psoriatic arthritis, and IBD. Reduced presence of beneficial species can lead to functional consequences, including impaired immune regulation at the gut level, which then has the potential to affect distant organ systems.

Another mechanism for gut microflora's involvement in the pathogenesis of psoriasis may be the penetration of gut microorganisms and their metabolites through the broken intestinal barrier into the systemic bloodstream. This has subsequent effects on distant organs, including skin and joints. The presence of gut microorganisms' DNA in the blood of psoriasis patients supports this hypothesis (Ramírez-Boscá A. et al., 2015).

1.3.2. Skin microbiome

The skin microbiome in psoriasis is peculiar. Compared to healthy skin, there is a decrease in alpha and beta diversity* and a change in species composition—a decrease in *Cutibacterium*, *Burkholderia spp.*, and *Lactobacilli* and an increase in *Corynebacterium kroppenstedii*, *Corynebacterium simulans*, *Neisseria spp.*, and *Finegoldia spp.* (**Table III-1-1**) (Olejniczak-Staruch I. et al., 2021). *S. aureus* and *Streptococcus pyogenes*, which stimulate the innate immune system, play a significant role in initiating and maintaining psoriasis.

These pathogens are present in increased numbers in psoriasis lesions. Enterotoxins produced by *S. aureus* play an essential role in the pathogenesis of the disease. Throat and nasal streptococcal infection, especially beta-hemolytic *S. pyogenes*, is responsible for guttate psoriasis and chronic plaque psoriasis. This bacterium carries streptococcal M protein and streptococcal peptidoglycan, which activate T cells. Streptococcal peptidoglycan binds to class II molecules

---

* Alpha diversity is the diversity of microbial species within the gut microbiome of the same individual. Beta diversity refers to differences in the species diversity of the gut microbiota between individuals.

of the major histocompatibility complex (MHC) and T-cell receptors, initiating a pathologic inflammatory response and cytokine release (Liang X. et al., 2021). Moreover, streptococcal M protein and pyrogenic exotoxins (A, B, and C) bind to dendritic cells, macrophages, and keratinocytes, activating T cells. T cells from people with psoriasis can simultaneously react with homologous peptides of streptococcal M-protein and keratins 6 and 17, contributing to the development of psoriasis.

Table III-1-1. Skin microbiome and cytokine profile alterations in psoriasis (Zhang X.E. et al., 2024)

INCREASED POPULATION	DECREASED POPULATION	CYTOKINES
Firmicutes	*Actinobacteria*	↑IL-1, ↑IL-6,
Streptococcus spp.	*Gordoniaceae*	↑ IL-8, ↑IL-17,
Prevotella	*Staphylococcus epidermidis*	↑IL-12, ↑IL-23,
Staphylococcus spp.	*Cutibacterium spp.*	↑IL-22, ↑TNFα,
Staphylococcus aureus	*Staphylococcus spp.*	↑IFN-α, ↑TGF-β,
Staphylococcus pettenkoferi	*Cutibacterium acnes*	↑iNOS, ↑HSP70
Staphylococcus sciuri	*Cutibacterium granulosum*	
Corynebacterium kroppenstedii	*Burkholderia spp.*	
Corynebacterium simulans	*Lactobacilli*	
Neisseria spp.		
Finegoldia spp.		

The epidermis's characteristic functional feature in psoriasis is the secretion of large amounts of antimicrobial peptides. However, this does not favor a healthy skin microbiome.

Thus, people with psoriasis lose another ally in the fight against the disease — a healthy microbiome, which not only repels the attacks of pathogenic microorganisms but also supports the self-tolerance of the immune system, preventing the fire of inflammation.

Chapter 2
Clinical presentation, diagnosis, and treatment

2.1. Clinical manifestation

2.1.1. Clinical types of psoriasis

- **Psoriasis vulgaris** is characterized by the appearance of pink–red papules with clear borders, with a tendency to merge and form plaques of various sizes and shapes, covered with silvery-white scales (**Fig. III-2-1**). The plaques are localized mainly on

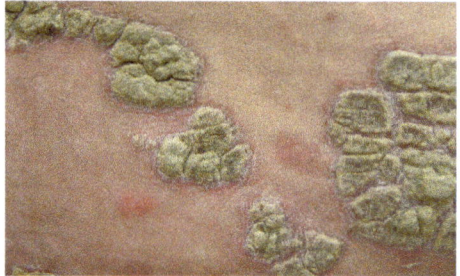

Figure III-2-1. Psoriatic plaque (adapted from Wikipedia)

the scalp, the extensor surface of the elbow and knee joints, the lumbar region, and the sacrum but may be located on other skin areas. Patients may be bothered by itching of varying degrees of intensity. The psoriatic triad characterizes the rashes.

- **Seborrheic psoriasis** is diagnosed when rashes are localized only on seborrheic areas of the skin (scalp, nasolabial and behind-the-ear folds, chest, and interscapular area). In seborrheic psoriasis, the scales are usually yellowish, the scaling on the head may be very severe, and the rash may extend from the scalp to the forehead, forming the so-called "psoriatic crown" (**Fig. III-2-2**).

- **Inverse psoriasis** — rashes are localized in places of natural skin folds (inguinal, gluteal, axillary, pectoral, posterior ear folds, on the extensor surfaces of the extremities). Cracks or furrows may form in the center or along the edges of the affected skin areas. There may be no desquamation (**Fig. III-2-3**).
- **Guttate psoriasis** is an acute form of the disease characterized by the appearance on the skin of numerous bright red drop-shaped papules 0.5–1.5 cm in diameter with slight desquamation and infiltration (**Fig. III-2-4**).
- **Pustular psoriasis** manifests as generalized or limited rashes, often located on the palms and soles, and is represented by superficial pustular elements (**Fig. III-2-5**).
- **Generalized pustular psoriasis (von Zumbusch)** manifests as extensive erythema with sterile pustules. The erythematous lesions tend to merge. The generalized form progresses severely, with fever and malaise.

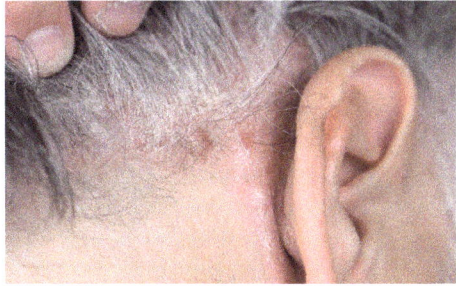

Figure III-2-2. Psoriasis of the scalp (adapted from Freepik)

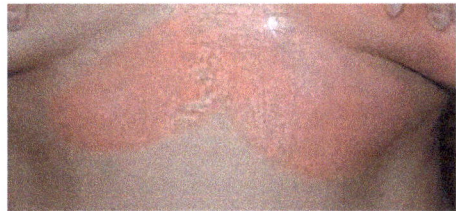

Figure III-2-3. Inverse psoriasis (adapted from Göblös A. et al., 2021)

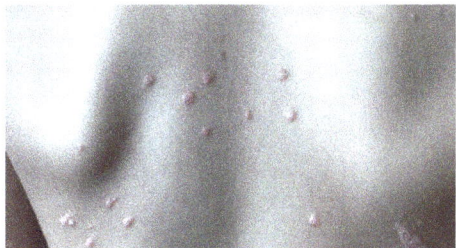

Figure III-2-4. Guttage psoriasis (9-years-old girl) (adapted from Wikipedia)

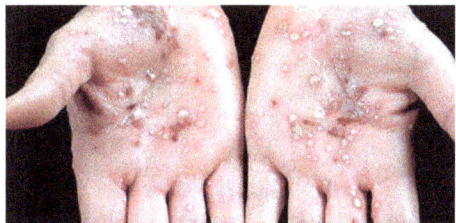

Figure III-2-5. Pustular psoriasis

- **Acrodermatitis continua of Hallopeau** — manifested by erythematous-squamous and vesiculopustular rashes on the distal phalanges of the fingers. Bright erythema, edema, and multiple pustules merging into "purulent lakes" are noted on the affected areas of the fingers.
- **Erythrodermic psoriasis** more often occurs when an existing psoriasis vulgaris is exacerbated by irritating factors or irrational treatment (bathing in the progressive stage, excessive insolation or UV overdose, use of permissive ointments in high concentrations during exacerbation). The skin becomes bright red, edematous, infiltrated, lichenified, and hot and is covered with many dry white scales that fall off easily when clothing is removed. Erythroderma covers more than 90% of the skin and is accompanied by itching, burning, and pain.
- **Psoriatic arthritis** — joint damage may develop simultaneously with or precede psoriatic skin rashes. Subsequently, there may be synchrony in developing exacerbations of psoriatic arthritis and skin lesions. The joint process is accompanied by reddening of the skin over the affected joints, swelling, pain, limitation of mobility, and morning stiffness. Joint deformities, ankyloses, enthesitis (inflammation of tendons in the area of their attachment to bones), dactylitis, and spondylitis may also be present.

2.1.2. Stages of psoriasis

In psoriasis, there is a staggered course of the disease.

- **The progressive stage (exacerbation)** is characterized by the appearance of new papules and plaques with an increase around the old ones (**Fig. III-2-6**), bright pink lesion coloration,

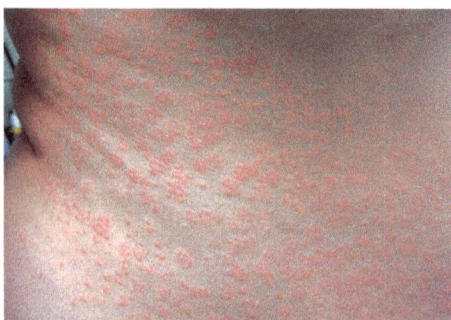

Figure III-2-6. Progressive stages of psoriasis: small bright pink papules merge into plaques (photo provided by V.I. Albanova)

and often itching. At this stage, the **Koebner phenomenon** — the appearance of new rashes on unaffected skin when it is traumatized — is observed.

- **Stationary stage (stabilization)** — new rashes do not appear, existing rashes do not increase in size, but also do not shrink, the color of rashes changes to stagnant-blue and dark red, lesions are covered with a large number of silvery-white scales (**Fig. III-2-7**), itching subsides.

- **Regressive stage (resolution)** — areas of healthy skin appear in the center of lesions, large lesions disintegrate into parts (**Fig. III-2-8**), and secondary pigmentation disorder is formed — more often decreased but sometimes increased (depending on the treatment performed).

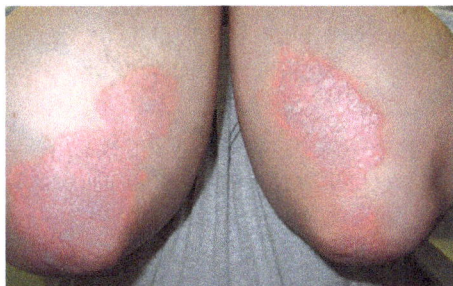

Figure III-2-7. Stationary stage of psoriasis (photo provided by V.I. Albanova)

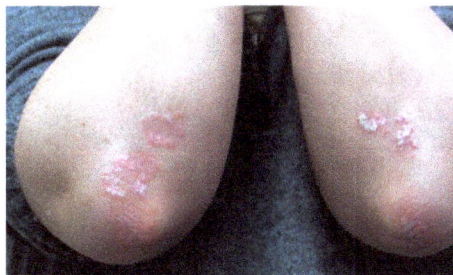

Figure III-2-8. Psoriasis in regression (photo provided by V.I. Albanova)

2.1.3. Seasonal variability

There is no universally recognized psoriasis classification related to seasonal influences, but this disease is often exacerbated in certain weather conditions. According to a literature review by Jensen K.K. et al. (2022), about 50% of psoriasis manifestations are not influenced by season, approximately 30% improve during summer, and about 20% do better in winter. In a small number of patients, the condition worsens significantly in summer. Season-dependent changes in psoriasis should be considered an individual patient characteristic that may determine the success of UVB/A therapy and provide a basis for recommending whether to sunbathe.

The effectiveness of insolation depends on the disease stage. In the progressive stage, sun exposure is fraught with deterioration, and in the regressive stage, patients can safely go to beach resorts. The stationary stage requires caution, as a rapid relapse is possible. Sun protection of the whole skin is necessary during retinoid treatment and phototherapy, for the summer form of psoriasis, and for external treatment with tar, retinoids, and calcipotriol. The degree of protection depends on the skin phototype. Patients should also be advised to refrain from sunbathing within the first month after treatment completion.

They should also be cautioned to prevent sunburns, which can cause a new exacerbation. Besides, the remaining light spots on the sites of resolved rashes on the background of dark tan become more noticeable. UV rays have an undesirable impact on hair because they cause photochemical destruction of the structure of the hair shaft.

Spa treatments for people with psoriasis are carried out at sea and balneological resorts at any time of the year during remission. In a circle of similar patients, they are unlikely to worry about the reaction of others to skin lesions. Swimming in the sea and pool, walking in the open air — all these activities favorably affect the patient's psychological status and contribute to the prolongation of remission.

2.2. Diagnostic criteria and differential diagnosis

The diagnosis of psoriasis is based on the clinical picture of the disease, the symptoms of the psoriatic triad, and the presence of the Koebner phenomenon in the progressive stage (**Fig. III-2-9**). In some cases, a histologic analysis of a tissue sample biopsied from the affected skin is performed to confirm the diagnosis.

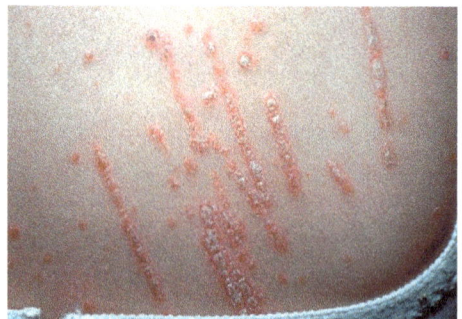

Figure III-2-9. Psoriatic rashes at skin scratching sites

Psoriatic triad — phenomena arising sequentially when scraping papular rashes: stearin spot (when lightly scraping the papule, there is an increase in scaling, giving the surface of the papules a resemblance to a rubbed drop of stearin); terminal film (the appearance after complete removal of scales — wet, thin, shiny, translucent surface of the elements); spot bleeding (the appearance after careful scraping of the terminal film of pinpoint, non-merging drops of blood).

The differential diagnosis of psoriasis should be made with:
- Papular rash in syphilis
- Lichen planus
- Pityriasis rosea (Zhiber's illness)
- Seborrheic eczema
- Atopic dermatitis
- Parapsoriasis
- Pytiriasis rubra pilaris

2.3. Treatment

Psoriasis requires long-term treatment. Even after the rashes completely resolve, subclinical inflammation may persist, eventually leading to disease recurrence in the exact location. Although long-term psoriasis treatment is paramount, this approach is still challenging in clinical practice (especially for mild and moderate forms). This is partly due to a lack of suitable treatments or patient refusal to follow recommendations owing to discomfort or social constraints experienced with topical/systemic agents. For these reasons, many patients do not receive appropriate treatment.

The therapeutic modalities for psoriasis should be based on its severity which should be assessed using the Psoriasis Area and Severity Index (PASI). The PASI represents a composite score of erythema (E), infiltration (I), scaling (S), and area (A) of the psoriatic plaque.

As the PASI scale is used to rate the severity of psoriatic lesions, it can be adopted to assess the patient's response to therapy. The PASI is the most frequently used system and widely used instrument in psoriasis trials. It combines the assessment of the severity of psoriatic lesions and the area affected into a single score, typically ranging from 0 (indicating no disease) to 72 (indicating maximal disease severity) (Bożek A., Reich A., 2017).

To assess the severity of psoriasis using the PASI, the body is divided into four regions: the head (h), upper extremities (u), trunk (t), and lower extremities (l), with each region representing a specific percentage of the total body surface area (BSA). These regions account for 10%, 20%, 30%, and 40% of the total BSA, respectively.

For each of these anatomical regions, healthcare providers assess the severity of psoriasis independently for erythema (redness), induration (thickness), and scaling using a scale that ranges from 0 (indicating no symptoms) to 4 (indicating very severe symptoms).

- **Induration:** Refers to the thickness or hardening of the psoriatic lesions.
- **Erythema:** Assesses the redness or inflammation associated with the psoriatic plaques.
- **Scaling:** Evaluates the extent of scaling of the skin affected by psoriasis.

The degree of psoriatic involvement in each region is classified into the following categories (**Fig. III-2-10**):

0 = No involvement
1 = Involvement of 1% to 9% of the area
2 = 10% to 29%
3 = 30% to 49%
4 = 50% to 69%
5 = 70% to 89%
6 = 90% to 100%

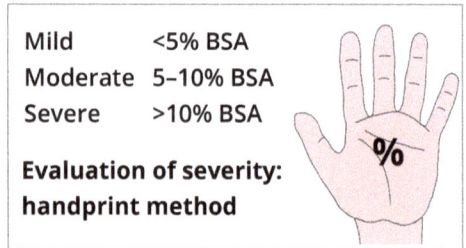

Mild   <5% BSA
Moderate   5–10% BSA
Severe   >10% BSA

Evaluation of severity: handprint method

%

Figure III-2-10. PASI determination using the palm

The PASI score is calculated using the following formula (**Fig. III-2-11**):

$$PASI = [0.1 \times (Eh + Ih + Sh) \times Ah] + [0.2 \times (Eu + Iu + Su) \times Au] + [0.3 \times (Et + It + St) \times At] + [0.4 \times (El + Il + Sl) \times Al]$$

where E — erythema, I — induration, S — scaling, A — area, h — head score, u — upper extremities score, t — trunk score, and l — lower extremities score.

Erythema severity in psoriatic lesions

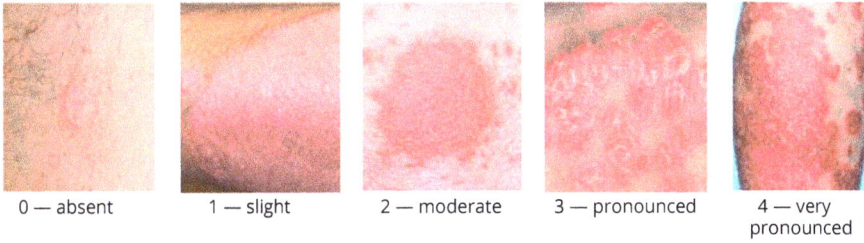

| 0 — absent | 1 — slight | 2 — moderate | 3 — pronounced | 4 — very pronounced |

Expression of infiltration in psoriatic lesions

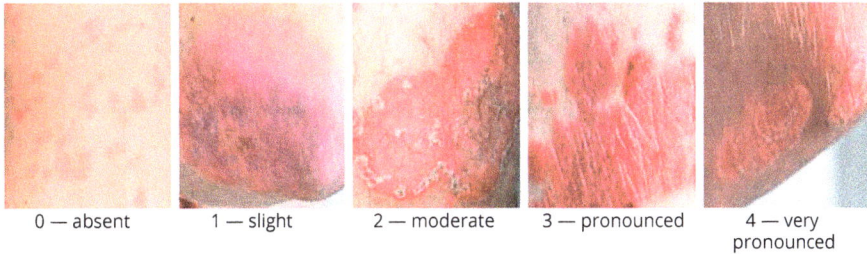

| 0 — absent | 1 — slight | 2 — moderate | 3 — pronounced | 4 — very pronounced |

Severity of desquamation in psoriatic lesions

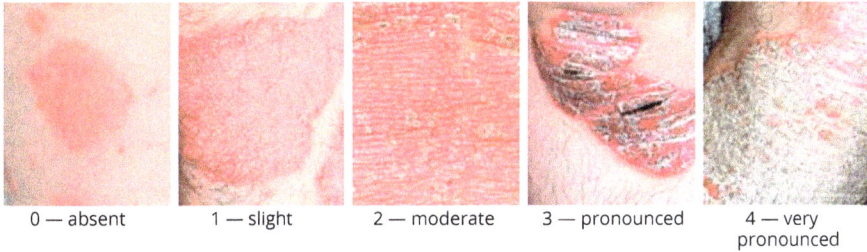

| 0 — absent | 1 — slight | 2 — moderate | 3 — pronounced | 4 — very pronounced |

Figure III-2-11. Assessment of the severity of clinical manifestations of psoriasis when calculating the PASI score (adapted from Kubanov A.A. et al., 2016)

This formula combines the individual scores for each region and aspect to provide an overall PASI score (from 0 to 72), which is a numerical representation of the severity of psoriasis, interpreted as follows:

- up to 9 points —mild
- 10–19 points — moderate
- 20–72 points — severe

2.3.1. Topical therapy

Topical therapy is usually the first-line treatment modality for all patients.

In patients with moderate to severe disease receiving systemic therapy or phototherapy, concomitant topical treatment is also indicated, as residual disease may significantly impact health-related quality of life.

The choice of topical agent should be based on the anatomical region affected by the rash and the nature and severity of clinical symptoms such as hyperkeratosis, redness, inflammation, pruritus, and pain (**Table III-2-1** and **III-2-2**).

Table III-2-1. Advantages, disadvantages, and practical recommendations for the use of different forms of topical agents (Thaçi D. et al., 2020)

PRODUCT	ADVANTAGES	DISADVANTAGES	APPLICATION
Ointment	• It is occlusive and improves penetration and efficiency • Moisturizing effect • Simple formula, often without preservatives	• Highly greasy, does not evaporate, poorly absorbed • Persists on the skin for long periods of time, which may be unacceptable to the patient	• Dry, thick, scaly plaques on the body • Not suitable for the scalp
Cream	• Less greasy, more easily spreadable than ointment, has some moisturizing effect • Does not impair the aesthetic characteristics of the skin	• Less pronounced occlusive effect, lower penetration and efficacy compared to ointment	• All areas of the body • With proper application technique, it can be used on the scalp

Continued on p. 175

PRODUCT	ADVANTAGES	DISADVANTAGES	APPLICATION
Water- or lipid-based gel	• Easy to apply, easy to spread • Does not impair the aesthetic characteristics of the skin	• Minimal or no occlusive effect • Minimal moisturizing properties	On all areas of the body, especially good for the scalp
Spray foam with water–alcohol or emollient base	• Easy to apply, easy to spread • Usually without preservatives • Some skin moisturizing if contains emollient • Does not degrade the aesthetic characteristics of the skin	• Minimal occlusive and moisturizing effect (water–alcohol base) • May increase skin oiliness (emollient base) Risk of burning, irritation and dry skin (water–alcohol base)	On all parts of the body, especially good for the scalp (except emollient-based products)
Lotion	• Easy to apply, non-greasy • Does not impair the aesthetic characteristics of the skin • It has a cooling effect	It has no occlusive effect; moisturizing effect is absent or weakly expressed	• Scalp • Not suitable for skin with thickened plaques
Alcoholic or aqueous solution	• Easy to apply, non-greasy, leaves no residue • Does not impair the aesthetic characteristics of the skin	• Burning, irritation, and dryness if the product is alcohol-based • Must be shaken (inhomogeneous solution)	• Scalp • Alcohol solutions should be avoided if they dry and damage the skin
Shampoo	• Designed for use on the scalp • Non-greasy	• Does not have occlusive and moisturizing effect • Short skin contact time	Scalp

Table III-2-2. Topical agent selection according to rash localization and estimated time needed to notice improvements (Thaçi D. et al., 2020)

AREA	THERAPEUTIC APPROACH	TIME NEEDED FOR IMPROVEMENT ONSET
Torso	• Vitamin D derivatives (dose should not exceed 5 mg per week) • Combination of vitamin D derivatives and corticosteroids • Strong or ultra-strong corticosteroids (short-term use only) • Salicylic acid + corticosteroids	2–4 weeks
Limbs	• Combination of vitamin D derivatives and corticosteroids • Strong or ultra-strong corticosteroids (short-term use only) • Salicylic acid + corticosteroids • Overnight occlusion at the beginning of treatment (polyethylene gloves or socks) • Propylene glycol + corticosteroids	4 weeks
Scalp	• Combination of vitamin D derivatives and corticosteroids • Strong or ultra-strong corticosteroids (short-term use only) • Salicylic acid + corticosteroids • Tar + salicylic acid + sulfur	4 weeks
Face	• Mild to moderate corticosteroids • Topical calcineurin inhibitors	2 weeks
Perianal or genital area and skin folds (axillary, inframammary, or inguinal)	• Mild to moderate corticosteroids • Topical calcineurin inhibitors	2 weeks

The key psoriasis symptoms (**Table III-2-3**) can also guide the type and form of topical agent choice.

Table III-2-3. Selection of topical agent according to clinical symptoms of the disease

DRUG	ERYTHEMA	SCALING	HYPERKERATOSIS, INFILTRATION	ITCHING
Corticosteroids	+++	+	++	++/+++
Vitamin D derivatives	+/++	+/++	+/++	—
CAL/BDP	+++	++	+++	+++
Topical calcineurin inhibitors	+/++	—	+	++
Salicylic acid	—	+++	—	—
Urea	—	++	—	+
Tar	+	+	++	++

"–" — no effect, "+" — light effect, "++" — moderate effect, "+++" — significant effect. CAL/DBP — calcipotriene/betamethasone dipropionate.

Satisfactory improvement (e.g., reduction in redness, scaling, plaque thickness, and size of the affected area) should be noticed within two weeks. Improvement in some symptoms, such as itching, may occur within a few days. After about four weeks, a marked improvement (complete or almost complete disappearance of the rash) should be expected. Suppose there is no clinically significant improvement after four weeks. In that case, the patient should be assessed for adherence to the recommendations, and treatment should be changed if, despite adherence, there is no improvement.

Recent evidence suggests that topical application of a combination of corticosteroids and vitamin D derivatives (calcipotriene/betamethasone dipropionate) is the most effective approach to psoriasis therapy and can be used for long-term treatment and to reduce relapse rates (Gerdes S. et al., 2024).

A combination of 50 µg/g calcipotriol and betamethasone dipropionate 0.5 mg/g in gel, ointment, foam, or emulsion (cream) form can be used. The drug has been approved as a starter for treating psoriasis in many countries, and according to recent publications, it outperforms other topical agents in terms of efficacy (Papp K.A. et al., 2022).

In 2022, the U.S. Food and Drug Administration (FDA) approved two new non-steroidal topical agents for treating plaque psoriasis: tapinarof cream 1% and roflumilast cream 0.3% (Bruno M. et al., 2023). Their significant advantages are their high safety profile and tolerability, the possibility of long-term use, and the lack of restrictions on the anatomical localization of rashes.

Tapinarof is a naturally occurring polyphenolic AhR-ligand that is believed to improve the course of psoriasis through immune modulation, normalization of the skin barrier, and reduction of oxidative stress. Specifically, *in vitro* studies show that tapinarof reduces the production of pro-inflammatory Th17 cytokines, increases the expression of skin barrier protein genes (filaggrin and loricrin), and reduces the activity of tissue-resident memory T cells, which are thought to contribute to recurrent psoriasis (**Fig. III-2-12**). Tapinarof also has antioxidant effects. The drug is indicated for use in adults and has no

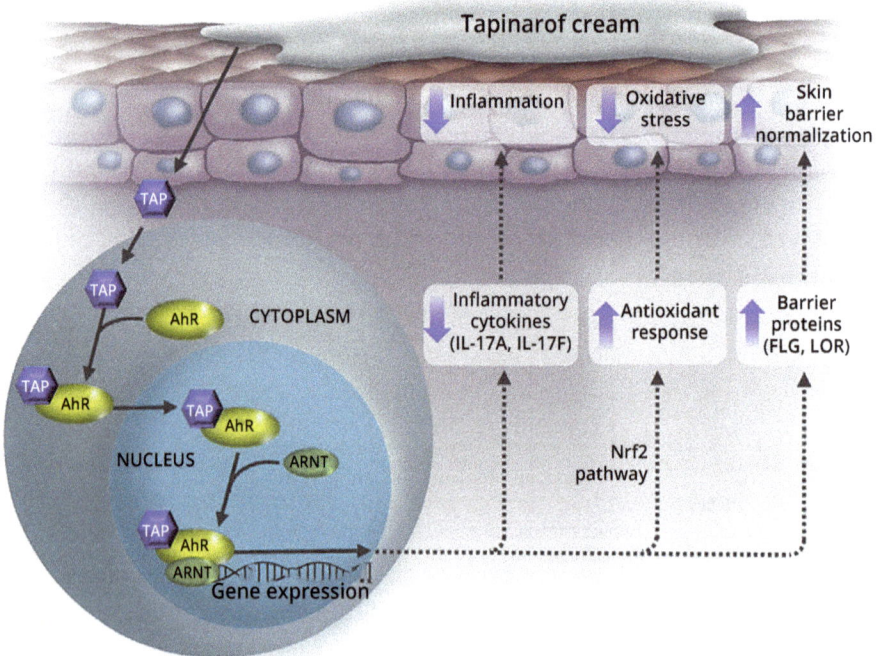

Figure III-2-12. Mechanisms of action of the AhR receptor modulator (tapinarof, TAP) in psoriasis (Bruno M. et al., 2023)

restrictions concerning psoriasis severity, anatomical localization, or duration of use.

Roflumilast belongs to selective inhibitors of PDE-4, a key enzyme involved in immune cell homeostasis. Increased PDE-4 activity in psoriasis lesions leads to an increase in pro-inflammatory mediators, making PDE-4 a suitable therapeutic target. Reducing pro-inflammatory mediator levels helps balance the immune response and normalize keratinocyte differentiation. Roflumilast is indicated for use in patients aged 12 years and older, with no restrictions regarding psoriasis severity, anatomical localization, or duration of use (O'Toole A., Gooderham M., 2023).

2.3.2. Systemic therapy

Systemic therapy is indicated for any psoriasis type in the following cases:
1. The disease cannot be controlled with topical therapy
2. Psoriasis has a significant impact on the patient's physical, psychological, or social well-being
3. If one or more of the following criteria are met:
   - Extensive rashes (e.g., more than 10% of the body surface is affected or the PASI score is greater than 10)
   - Psoriasis is associated with significant functional impairment and/or high levels of distress (e.g., severe nail disease)
   - Phototherapy has been ineffective, cannot be used, or has resulted in rapid relapse (defined as a recurrence of rashes with a severity at least 50% higher than the baseline in the previous three months) (NICE Clinical Guidelines, No. 153, 2017)

Immunosuppressive agents (cyclosporine, methotrexate, acitretin) and agents obtained using biotechnological methods (genetically engineered biological drugs) are used for systemic psoriasis therapy. The latter include TNFα inhibitors (adalimumab, infliximab, certolizumab pegol, etanercept), IL-17 inhibitors (ixekizumab, secukinumab), IL-12/23 inhibitors (ustekinumab), and IL-23 inhibitors (guselkumab) (Alzahrani S.A. et al., 2023).

2.4. Vitamin D and its analogs in psoriasis therapy

In an extensive meta-analysis of 19 studies with about 1,387 patients and 6,939 healthy controls, the vitamin D levels in psoriasis patients were compared to those of healthy study participants. The authors found significantly lower vitamin D levels (<20 UI) in patients with psoriasis (Moosazadeh M. et al., 2023). Higher levels of 25(OH) D — the prohormonal form of vitamin D, calcidiol — are associated with lesser severity of psoriasis manifestations (Disphanurat W. et al., 2019). Deficiency in psoriasis and psoriatic arthritis is seasonal — 80% of 145 subjects in the study conducted by Gisondi P. et al. (2012) had a deficiency in winter and 50% in summer.

Vitamin D deficiency can be caused by insufficient sun exposure (avoiding insolation, living in areas with low insolation, and unnecessarily using sunscreen with very high SPF), impaired vitamin D metabolism (intestinal, gallbladder, liver, and kidney diseases), old age (vitamin D synthesis slowdown), obesity (deposition of vitamin D in adipose tissue), pregnancy, lactation (increased vitamin D requirements), and long-term use of some drugs (anticonvulsants, GCSs, and antifungals for HIV treatment).

Vitamin D deficiency can be compensated by active insolation, consumption of vitamin D-containing or vitamin D-enriched foods, food supplements, and drugs.

2.4.1. Oral administration of vitamin D

Treatment of psoriasis by oral administration of vitamin D has been attempted as a part of several studies. Kamangar F. et al. (2013) failed to establish a clinical effect. Still, they noted a risk of increased blood calcium levels when high doses of vitamin D were used, cautioning that the calcium level in blood and urine during oral vitamin D administration should be carefully monitored. As a part of their investigation involving nine people with psoriasis, Finamor D.C. et al. (2013) found that oral vitamin D intake in high doses (35,000 IU per day) for six months in combination with a diet low in calcium (exclusion from the diet or reducing the proportion of dairy products and foods containing high levels of calcium, such as oatmeal and rice cereals, soy "milk"), while drinking 2.5 liters of water per day, led to a significant reduction in the PASI score without any side effects. The treatment regimen used by Disphanurat W. et al. (2019) — 23 patients received 60,000 IU of ergocalciferol (vitamin D2) at 2-week intervals for six months — led to a 35% and 43% decline in the PASI value after 3 and 6 months, respectively, compared to the baseline, which was a significantly greater reduction than in the placebo group. Lourencetti M. and Abreu M.M. (2018) found that oral administration of active vitamin D metabolites at 0.25–2 µg is effective and safe in psoriasis. In an earlier study conducted by Perez A. et al. (1996), treatment with calcitriol resulted in improvement in 88% of the study sample (26.5%, 36.2%, and 25.3% of the 85 participating patients had complete, moderate, and slight effects, respectively), with a change in creatinine metabolism without impairment of renal function. However, in several publications, opposite results are reported. For instance, a meta-analysis of four peer-reviewed studies with 333 patients examining the efficacy and safety of vitamin D intake in psoriasis showed no statistically significant effect of vitamin D intake on the severity of clinical manifestations of psoriasis according to the PASI (Dai Q. et al., 2023).

Despite these conflicting results, it is worth noting that Moosazadeh M. et al. (2023) recently established that systemic vitamin D supplementation can improve the skin condition in individuals with low 25(OH)D levels in the blood. This is particularly relevant since most psoriasis patients are vitamin D deficient. Thus, the favorable effect of vitamin D on the clinical manifestations of comorbidities, particularly metabolic syndrome and cardiovascular disease, should also be considered.

2.4.2. Topical application of vitamin D analogs

Topical application of the synthetic vitamin D analog — calcipotriol — proved safer and more effective. The effectiveness of external preparations is associated primarily with antiproliferative and anti-inflammatory properties, regulation of keratinocyte differentiation and apoptosis, and influence on immune processes in the skin. All these effects are realized through hormonal nuclear vitamin D receptors found in keratinocytes and fibroblasts. Moreover, keratinocytes themselves can produce the hormonally active form of vitamin D.

When applied topically, a decrease in keratinocyte proliferation and their improved differentiation, as well as reduced pro-inflammatory cytokine levels in the dermis were recorded by Nagpal S. et al. (2005). These authors also found that the positive effect on keratinocyte differentiation simultaneously caused the improvement of epidermal barrier properties, including the proper formation of the cornified envelopes.

In another study, topical calcipotriol ointment and gel were more effective than cream (Queille-Roussel C. et al., 2012). According to Lebwohl M. et al. (2007), an ointment application's most common side effects are discomfort, itching, erythema, and burning. Skin irritation was observed in approximately 20% of patients. In general, calcipotriol treatment is recognized as safe and effective, as side effects are mild and limited to the application site, due to which calcipotriol is included in many clinical guidelines (Arnone M. et al., 2019).

Management of vitamin D deficiency by administering topical and systemic dosage forms of the vitamin and its analogs appears to be important in preventing new exacerbations of psoriasis and maintaining a more favorable disease course.

2.5. Phototherapy

In most cases, psoriatic lesions on the skin are subjected to local treatment (Parrish J.A., Jaenicke K.F., 1981; Drew G.S., 2009). The main drawback of such regimens is the need to regularly apply medications to the skin, which is not always convenient and reduces compliance (De Arruda L.H., De Moraes A.P., 2001; Krueger G. et al., 2001). At the same time, as psoriasis therapy is carried out throughout life, undesirable adverse reactions, including those of a systemic nature, may be observed, negatively affecting patients' adherence to treatment. Thus, the search for new ways of psoriasis treatment continues, and phototherapy is considered one of the most promising directions.

The following wavelengths are used for psoriasis phototherapy:
- Broadband radiation in the 280–320 nm range (UVB)
- Narrowband radiation of 311 nm (Narrowband UVB Light Therapy, nbUVB)
- Long-wave radiation of 320–400 nm (UVA) is used with specific chemicals that increase the skin's sensitivity to UV

UV radiation of 311 nm wavelength (nbUVB) has the most significant clinical efficacy and safety, as well as several very significant advantages:
- Individual dose selection depending on skin phototype
- Almost no adverse effects
- When included in complex therapy, it leads to the complete resolution of the pathological process
- No need to use special photosensitizers before the session
- Significantly reduced likelihood of carcinogenesis
- It is not necessary to apply protective creams after the session
- Reduces the overall radiation exposure
- Preventive effect on healthy skin areas
- Relatively small list of contraindications

A significant advantage of phototherapy is that it is a convenient treatment mode — three sessions/week are carried out at the beginning, and the frequency is gradually decreased to one session/week. The sessions last from a few seconds to a few minutes, and 25–30 are usually sufficient to achieve persistent remission and significant symptom relief. Given the statistical data and many years of experience in using phototherapy in treating psoriasis worldwide, nbUVB therapy can be provided even to patients with small lesions on the knees and elbows without inflammation.

Other light-assisted treatments should not be used during phototherapy. Injections, hygienic facial cleansing, electrostimulation, and surgical interventions should be postponed until remission or used cautiously in the regressive period. It is worth considering that, even in the remission period, aesthetic injections, vaccinations, tattooing, peeling, mesotherapy, microneedling, fractional photothermolysis, and surgical interventions (especially those accompanied by painful sensations and experiences) can become a trigger for a new exacerbation.

2.5.1. IPL therapy

IPL systems use incoherent light radiation in the 500–1,200 nm wavelength range. In addition to the light source, the device includes an internal filter and several external (cutoff) filters, allowing the required wavelength to be selected. Thus, therapy based on selective photothermolysis with non-coherent polychromatic light can be delivered.

Contraindications to IPL treatment:

- Fresh tanning
- Darker skin phototypes (with caution)
- Taking photosensitizing antibiotics (doxycycline, minocycline)
- History of adverse reactions to IPL
- Menstruation

Safe use of laser and IPL requires appropriate personnel qualifications and competent patient selection. However, even under these conditions, side effects and complications (such as erythema, edema, purpura, and discoloration of target vessels) may still occur.

To reduce the likelihood of adverse events, the procedure should be postponed until the erythema disappears completely, aggressive cosmetics should not be applied to the affected area, and the patient should refrain from hot baths and Jacuzzis, as well as physical treatments that cause heavy sweating, insolation, and taking nonsteroidal anti-inflammatory drugs (NSAIDs). If the swelling is severe, a diuretic may be taken once a day.

- Possible post-treatment complications:
- Post-inflammatory hyperpigmentation
- Chessboard-pattern-like dyschromia
- Permanent scarring
- Epidermal burns

2.5.2. Laser therapy

Laser therapy is a relatively new psoriasis treatment modality, but the following benefits have already been observed:

- Ability to precisely target rashes without affecting the intact skin surrounding them, minimizing the photodamaging and carcinogenic effects, as well as the risk of adverse reactions
- Lack of significant systemic effects, making it suitable for children and patients with contraindications to other therapeutic methods
- Comfortable regimen — limited number of sessions, short session time, and long inter-session intervals
- Accessibility and convenience in treating lesions of any localization, including scalp, inverse, palm, and plantar forms of psoriasis, as well as nail lesions
- Possibility of use as an alternative in case of low effectiveness of drug therapy or patient's refusal to take medication
- In most cases, visible positive dynamics and a long remission period are quickly achieved
- Possibility of combining with local therapy to potentiate the therapeutic effect

Unfortunately, **laser therapy is effective only in chronic skin lesions with a torpid stable course and limited lesion area (up to 10%)**, which is the main indication for its use. The use of laser radiation in patients with an unstable disease course and those in the progressive stage of the disease is currently considered inappropriate.

A variety of laser treatments for psoriasis are presently available (**Table III-2-1**):

- Localized excimer laser irradiation
- Selective vascular coagulation
- Spatially modulated ablation
- Laser ablation

Local excimer laser therapy

The excimer laser in quasi-continuous mode* generates radiation with a wavelength of 308 nm, which belongs to the UVB part of the spectrum. The radiation is transmitted through a fiber-optic conductor to the lesion area, allowing localized treatment without affecting healthy skin.

---

* Quasi-continuous mode is a mode of light-emitting diode (LED) operation in which the LED is turned on at short enough intervals to reduce thermal effects significantly but long enough to consider its operation nearly continuous.

Table III-2-1. Laser treatment of psoriasis: clinical efficacy, and possible complications

	LOCAL LASER IRRADIATION	SELECTIVE VASCULAR COAGULATION	SPATIALLY MODULATED ABLATION
Radiation	Excimer laser (308 nm)	• PDL (585, 595 nm) • Nd:YAG/KTP (532 nm)	Er:YAG (2940 nm) with SMA module
Indications	• Plaque psoriasis • Inverse psoriasis • Psoriasis of the scalp • Palmoplantar psoriasis • Nail psoriasis	• Plaque psoriasis • Inverse psoriasis • Palmoplantar psoriasis • Nail psoriasis	• Plaque psoriasis • Inverse psoriasis • Psoriasis of the scalp • Palmoplantar psoriasis
Therapeutic course	4–10 or more sessions, twice per week, cumulative dose should be monitored	5–7 sessions, 1 session/2–3 weeks	1–7 sessions, 1 session or more/3–4 weeks
Clinical improvement	Improvement of varying degrees up to complete disappearance of rashes		
Maximum remission duration	Up to 2 years	Up to 3 years	Approx. 3 years
Complications	Blisters, erosions, hyperpigmentation	Blisters, erosions, dyschromia	None have been noted

SMA — spatially modulated ablation; Er:YAG — erbium-doped yttrium-aluminum-garnet laser; Nd:YAG/KTP — neodymium-doped yttrium-aluminum-garnet / potassium-titanyl-phosphate laser

The mechanism of action of laser and non-laser (excimer lamp) sources of UVB radiation is the same — they suppress keratinocyte proliferation and induce apoptosis of pro-inflammatory T cells (Furuhashi T. et al., 2011; Mudigonda T. et al., 2012a, 2012b). However, psoriatic plaques can tolerate a much higher dose of radiation than normal skin, which non-laser light sources cannot provide — this is what a high-energy collimated light-emitting device (laser) is for.

Available empirical data show that T-cell apoptosis is more active under excimer laser irradiation than traditional nbUVB phototherapy. Thus, as excimer laser is more aggressive than conventional UV phototherapy while facilitating localized delivery, the efficiency of each session is increased. This accelerates plaque clearance, reduces the number of procedures and course duration, and lessens the risk of adverse reactions (**Fig. III-2-13**) (Feldman S.R. et al., 2002; Hong J. et al., 2007; Gattu S. et al., 2010).

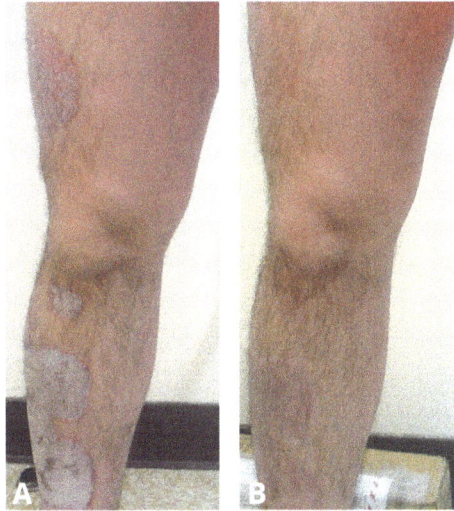

Figure III-2-13. Treatment of plaque psoriasis with an excimer laser at a wavelength of 308 nm: A — before treatment; B — 3 months after the last session (21 sessions in total) (adapted from Park K.K. et al., 2012)

In practice, two therapeutic approaches are utilized:

1. Exposure to **high doses of radiation (8–16 minimal erythema doses, MED)** allows for the achievement of faster positive dynamics and remission with a pronounced recovery period, albeit at an increased risk of phototoxic reactions.

2. Exposure to **low (0.5–1 MED)** and **medium doses (2–6 MED)** with a gradual increase — the duration of such a course is longer, but the severity of post-procedural changes and the risk of adverse reactions is lower.

Treatment is carried out in two sessions/week for 2–4 weeks; patients tolerate the procedures well and do not require anesthesia. According to Feldman S.R. et al. (2002), during excimer laser treatment (with 10 sessions on average), the PASI value can be reduced by 75–90%. The effectiveness of excimer laser in treating psoriasis of the scalp and nails has also been reported (Taylor C.R., Racette A.L., 2004; Morison W.L. et al., 2006).

Adverse reactions, such as itching, blisters, erosions, and hyperpigmentation, may occur, but no cases of scarring have been documented. It should, however, be noted that prolonged exposure to excimer laser radiation can cause DNA mutations, activation of oncogenes, reduced immune surveillance, and, as a consequence, the appearance of malignant skin tumors (squamous cell cancer and melanoma) (Taneja A. et al., 2003). It has been noted that treatment of psoriasis with 308-nm excimer laser in combination with external application of drugs (calcipotriol, anthralin, retinoids) can improve therapeutic efficacy and reduce the cumulative dose of UV irradiation, thereby reducing the risk of carcinogenesis (Debbaneh M.G. et al., 2015).

Selective vascular coagulation

Dilation and proliferation of dermal papillary vessels support local inflammation in psoriasis lesions. Endothelial changes are a therapeutic target for selective vascular coagulation, which aims to "cauterize" dilated capillaries. Subsequently, pro-inflammatory T-cell migration into tissues and mediator expression are reduced.

Pulsed dye lasers (PDLs) operating at 585 and 595 nm can be used for selective vascular coagulation, as different types of hemoglobin effectively absorb their yellow–green radiation.

Studies on treating psoriasis with PDL indicate 57–82% positive responses to therapy, with remission of about 15 months (Taibjee S.M. et al., 2005).

Zelickson B.D. et al. (1996) studied clinical and histological changes in the skin of psoriasis patients treated with PDL and observed significant improvement when both short (450 μs) and long (1500 μs) PDL pulses were used. In palmoplantar and nail psoriasis, PDL therapy leads to reasonable patient satisfaction. It can be combined with topical drugs to increase effectiveness (De Leeuw J. et al., 2006; Fernández-Guarino M. et al., 2009; Oram Y. et al., 2010; Al-Mutairi A., Elkashlan M., 2013).

Comparative studies of PDL and excimer laser efficacy indicate that the latter is superior in psoriasis therapy. At the same time, PLD requires fewer sessions and is less likely to cause undesirable side effects. Moreover, some patients with abnormal microcirculation of psoriatic plaques who are insensitive to excimer laser radiation respond well to PDL (Hruza G.J., 2005; Taibjee S.M. et al., 2005).

As a part of their study, De Leeuw J. et al. (2009) compared the PDL and excimer laser effectiveness and looked for synergies between the two treatment modalities. No significant differences were found between PDL and excimer laser, and no synergism was observed, suggesting that combining these treatment modalities does not increase the effectiveness of this approach and has no grounds for application.

In psoriasis, PDL therapy is carried out through 2–7 sessions with an interval of 2–3 weeks, which is usually sufficient to achieve clinical results. Procedures are well tolerated and do not require anesthesia. In the area of exposure, swelling, darkening of color, and purpura formation may occur after treatment — these phenomena persist for 7–10 days with gradual resolution. Positive effects manifest in a notable reduction in infiltration, erythema, desquamation, and psoriatic lesion area. If the radiation energy is too high, blisters and erosions in the treated area may form.

Laser-induced vascular complications are rare, but hyperpigmentation or scar formation is possible if the recommended energy parameters are exceeded.

Spatially modulated ablation (SMA)

This treatment modality requires an Er:YAG laser equipped with an SMA module, consisting of a lens system that allows redistribution of the energy flow in the light spot with alternation of its maxima and minima, each of 50 µm duration.

SMA's action on the skin is based on the photoacoustic (photomechanical) effect. This mechanism is realized when a massive amount of energy is transferred to the chromophore (water) over a very short interval (in the ns and ps range). Such high-energy ultra-short pulses cause electrons to detach from chromophores, forming a rapidly expanding plasma cloud that eventually "explodes" with the formation of shockwaves. This is believed to lead to the formation of "optical breakdowns" accompanied by cavitation (forming cavities of 0.1–0.2 mm diameter) without residual thermal damage.

The photoacoustic effect is characteristic of picosecond lasers. It also appears when Er:YAG is operated in a special mode in which optical energy is converted into a mechanical wave propagating deep into the tissue. This transformation is called spatially modulated ablation (SMA) and is performed by the SMA module (Volkova N.V. et al., 2017). With its help, the light beam is scattered and causes microablation dots. The resulting acoustic waves propagate through the tissues to a depth of up to 6 mm, forming microshock and microdestruction areas with minimal skin surface damage. Microdamage in the skin's deep layers triggers regeneration, leading to remodeling of the dermis structure. Er:YAG/SMA can be used for skin rejuvenation and scar revision, providing a safer alternative to fractional CO_2 laser.

The mechanism of the photoacoustic impact in psoriatic lesions has yet to be studied. The treatment results in antiproliferative and anti-inflammatory effects. Consequently, the typical layer-by-layer structure of the epidermis is gradually restored, along with the elimination of hyperkeratosis, inflammatory dermal infiltration, and abnormal changes in the microcirculatory papillary network.

In the experiments conducted by Kalashnikova N.G. (2014), a positive clinical response was obtained in 97% of plaque cases (**Fig. III-2-14**), inverse forms of psoriasis (**Fig. III-2-15**), and 81% of scalp psoriasis cases (**Fig. III-2-16**). The author also demonstrated promising results in palmoplantar forms of psoriasis (**Fig. III-2-17**). However, further study

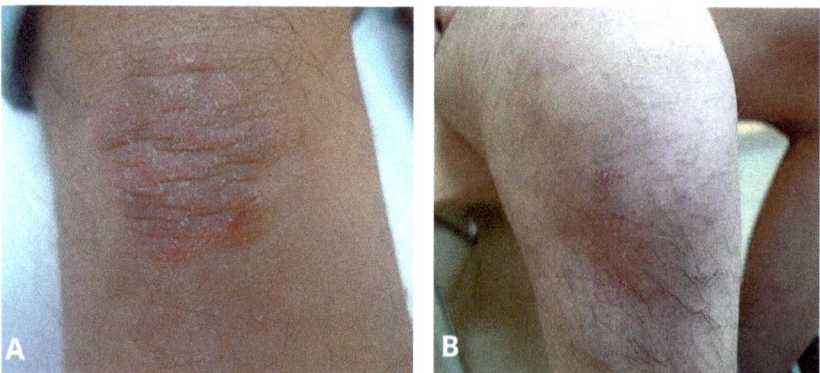

Figure III-2-14. Treatment of plaque psoriasis Er:YAG/SMA: A — before treatment; B — 2 months after the last session (3 sessions in total) (photo provided by N.G. Kalashnikova and D.S. Urakova)

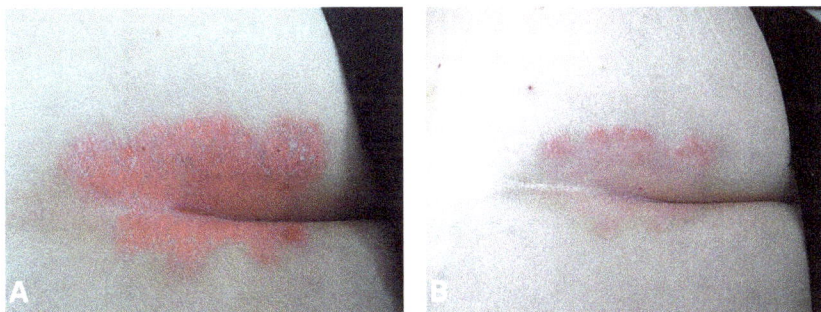

Figure III-2-15. Treatment of inverse psoriasis with Er:YAG/SMA: A — before treatment; B — 3 weeks after a single session (photo provided by N.G. Kalashnikova and D.S. Urakova)

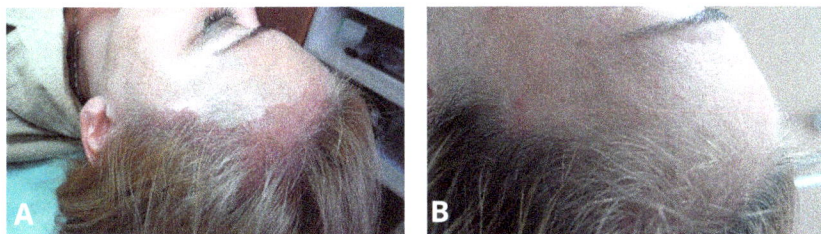

Figure III-2-16. Treatment of scalp psoriasis with Er:YAG/SMA: A — before treatment; B — 4 months after the last session (7 sessions in total) (photo provided by N.G. Kalashnikova and D.S. Urakova)

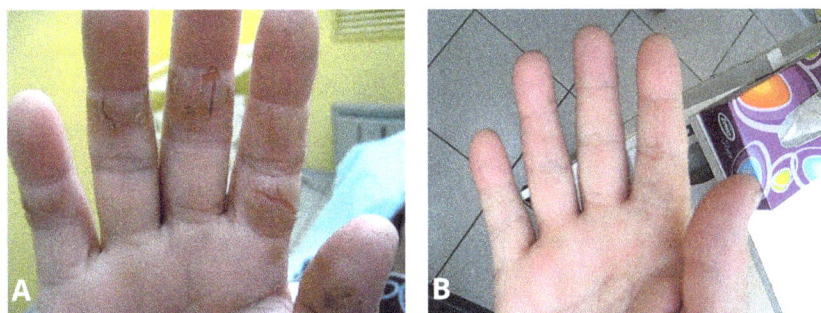

Figure III-2-17. Treatment of palmoplantar psoriasis with Er:YAG/SMA: A — before treatment; B — 1.5 months after the last session (2 sessions in total) (photo provided by N.G. Kalashnikova and D.S. Urakova)

is required to confirm these findings due to the small number of patients involved in this investigation.

Psoriasis treatment based on SMA is carried out in 1–10 sessions (on average, 2.7 are required) with an interval of 3–4 weeks. The procedures are well tolerated and do not require anesthesia. The energy density (2–4 J/cm^2) depends on the severity of peeling (the higher the degree, the higher the parameter settings). In the post-session period, crust formation with subsequent exfoliation is noted after 5–7 days. Visual positive dynamics in the form of plaque clearing, reduction of erythema, and infiltration are observed by the end of the 2nd week and reach the maximum by the 3–4th week without any complications (Kalashnikova N.G., 2014).

Laser ablation

Laser ablation was the first laser treatment of psoriatic lesions. It was performed in 1986 and has since become more prevalent, whereby two types of laser devices are presently used:
1. Carbon dioxide (CO_2) laser of 10,600 nm wavelength
2. Er:YAG laser of 2940 nm wavelength

These lasers target water as their primary chromophore. High absorption coefficient of water ensures the realization of a photothermal effect through the evaporation of superficial skin layers. Treating the lesion in several passes, the number of which depends on the type of laser radiation and the severity of the hyperkeratosis, helps clear the skin of pathological tissues.

Achievement of clinical effect after a single session is possible, with the removal of the epidermis and papillary layer of the dermis, resulting in the **reverse Koebner phenomenon** (disappearance of rashes and prolonged remission) — presumably due to a decrease in proinflammatory cells and mediator levels (Goldberg D.J., 2005).

This procedure is traumatic and requires preliminary anesthesia. It is characterized by a long recovery— lasting from 2 to 6 weeks, depending on the localization of the process — and the need for careful wound care.

Indications: single small plaques with stable torpid course and ineffective local treatment (Alora M.B. et al., 1998). At present, this method is not widely used.

Complications: infection, skin dyschromia, prolonged erythema, and scarring (including a pathological scenario involving the formation of hypertrophic scars).

Laser therapy is not a first-line treatment for psoriasis. Still, it is suitable for patients with a stable disease course whose affected area is limited in size, especially when traditional drug therapy is ineffective or the patient refuses it. Further studies in this direction seem interesting and promising.

Chapter 3
Basic skincare for psoriasis

3.1. Skin cleansing

When choosing a cleanser for skin affected by psoriasis, preference should be given to mild cleansers designed for sensitive skin, such as syndet soaps or gels with lipids and oils that maintain skin acidity in the physiological range. Cleansers used for atopic dermatitis can serve as a reference point.

Many patients prefer baby soap as the "most harmless" soap for washing. Unfortunately, baby soap dries the skin like other natural soaps with an alkaline pH (9 to 11). Perfumed soaps and gels are also undesirable, as some can irritate sensitive skin. Mild, odorless hygiene products are the best.

Cleansers do not have to be applied daily to the entire skin, but the affected areas should always be washed thoroughly to remove ointment residues. The same applies to sweaty and dirty skin, but if there is no dirt on the skin, it is sometimes better to rinse it with water.

In stationary and regressive stages, hyperkeratosis can be washed using a soft washcloth and gentle rubbing with a towel; taking salt baths 2–4 times a week has exfoliating and antipruritic effects.

In the acute stage, it is necessary to avoid skin-damaging manipulations, and after a shower, it is better to blot the skin gently. Light creams known as body milk or lotion are applied to slightly damp skin. They are low in fat and can be easily distributed over the skin, so their application to the entire body surface will take no more than a minute. The skin mustn't be displaced and should not be massaged (in the progressive stage, any additional irritation can provoke the appearance of new rashes like the Koebner phenomenon). On the driest areas (the front surface of the shins, sacrum, forearms, and shoulders), it is acceptable to apply a greasy (but not too thick!) cream or balm; on wet skin, body oil is preferable.

Generally, when psoriasis is advanced, it is better to shower with warm water rather than bathe. Any washing removes sebum, which forms a natural protective film and prevents the skin from drying out. Prolonged exposure to hot showers or baths improves blood circulation in the upper layers of the skin but also increases redness, itching, and scaling.

3.2. The healing effects of salt baths for psoriasis

Bathing in the sea and some mineral springs promotes healing and improves skin condition, especially dry skin. The clinical effects of a saline solution are based on several mechanisms.

First, the saline solution should be **hypertonic**; the concentration of dissolved salts and minerals in it should be higher than in the intercellular fluid and cytoplasm of living cells. Only in this case can its application yield favorable outcomes.

Second, the *stratum corneum* and living layers of the epidermis respond differently to the hypertonic solution due to their differences in structure and mechanisms for regulating water balance.

Third, the quality of the saline solution and its pH are essential.

3.2.1. Osmotic effects

Saline solutions have effects on the skin based on osmotic processes. In this case, it is necessary to distinguish the impacts related to the *stratum corneum* from those induced by processes in living skin layers.

Osmotic humidification of the *stratum corneum*
The intact *stratum corneum* is impermeable to water and water-soluble substances. When it comes into contact with a saline solution, water evaporates, leaving sediment on its surface. This phenomenon can

be observed after bathing in the sea. If we don't rinse with fresh water, once seawater evaporates, whitish streaks containing substances dissolved in seawater that didn't evaporate with it will be readily apparent on the skin.

However, if the *stratum corneum* is exposed to a salt solution for a long time (for example, during extended bathing), some dissolved molecules will penetrate it. In this case, salt ions enter corneocytes by simple diffusion along a concentration gradient — from the area where the concentration is higher (intercellular space) to the location where it is lower (inside corneocytes). The diffusion of salts will be accompanied by water movement into the corneocytes. The spontaneous transfer (diffusion) of a solvent through a semipermeable membrane into a more concentrated solution is called **osmosis**.

These processes increase the amount of water inside the corneocyte, which swells. **The mechanism of osmotic corneocyte swelling underlies the moisturizing effect of *stratum corneum***, which persists for quite a long time (up to several days if the skin is not washed) after bathing in seawater.

In the natural state, the water level inside the corneocytes is maintained by hygroscopic substances — high-molecular-weight keratin and low-molecular-weight NMF components. These substances retain water through ionic bonds, and the amount of water inside the corneocytes is directly related to the number of hygroscopic substances. If the amount of NMF declines (seen in the skin of AD and psoriasis patients, postmenopausal women, and infants), the water level in the corneocytes decreases, and they lose plasticity and become stiffer and more brittle. In this case, bathing in saline solutions will significantly help the skin — as the *stratum corneum* will be well moisturized.

Osmotic stimulation of epidermal cells

If the *stratum corneum* is intact, the salt components will not be able to reach the living cells. But if there are cracks in the barrier or its structure is broken as a result of disease (as, for example, in the area of psoriatic plaque), the salt solution will get under the *stratum corneum* and will mix with intercellular fluid, and living cells will be in a more concentrated (hypertonic) environment than usual. As a result, salt ions will

Hypotonic solution	Hypertonic solution	Isotonic solution

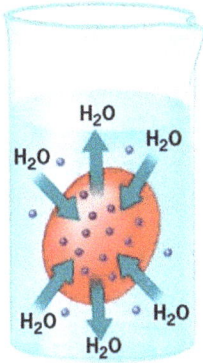

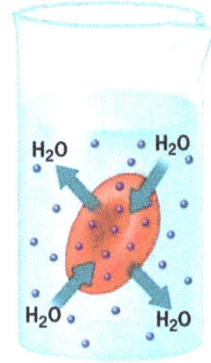

Net water gain
Cell swells

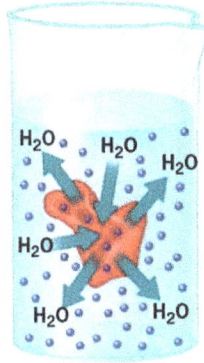

Net water loss
Cell shrinks

No net loss or gain

Figure III-3-1. Direction of water and ion flux through the cell membrane as a function of ambient osmolarity

enter the cell along the concentration gradient so that the cell will fill with water and swell. In an opposite scenario in which the cells are exposed to a less concentrated (hypotonic) solution, the flow of ions and water will be directed outward, and the cells will shrivel (**Fig. III-3-1**).

Unlike dead corneocytes, which do not react in any way to changes in their volume, living cells are susceptible to such fluctuations. Any volume change — upward (swelling) or downward (shriveling) — is a stimulus for cells to start compensatory reactions to return to their standard size. In the early stages of cell adaptation to hypo- or hypertonic conditions, inorganic ions and cell membrane ion channels play an essential role, including Na^+/K^+-ATPase, which controls the entry into and exit from the cell of sodium and potassium ions, Na^+/K^+-exchangers involved in maintaining the pH of the cytoplasm, etc. (**Fig. III-3-2**). Later, organic osmolytes — low-molecular-weight substances that regulate the osmotic pressure and viscosity of the cytoplasm within the cell — are "activated." Such substances include sugars (trehalose), polyols (glycerol, inositol, sorbitol), free amino acids (glycine, taurine, etc.), and methylamine (betaine). When the cell swells in a hypertonic environment, membrane channels open and allow the exit of osmolytes, which carry water out of the cell and maintain its normal volume.

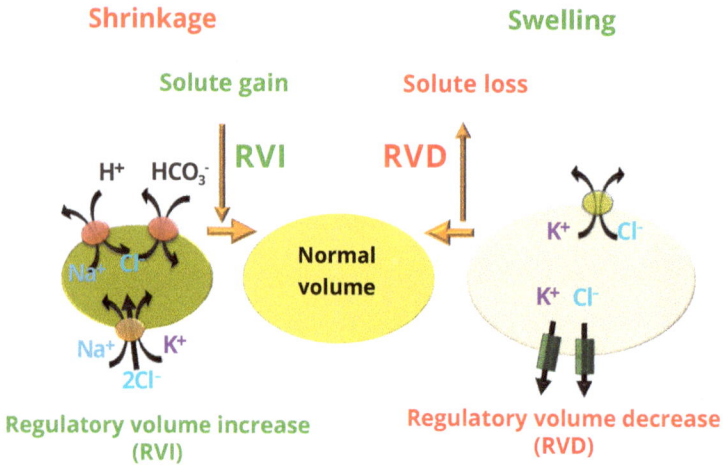

Figure III-3-2. Compensatory mechanisms enabling early cell adaptation to hypotonic and hypertonic environments (adapted from Carbajo J.M., Maraver F., 2018)

In addition to compensatory reactions aimed at volume maintenance, various biochemical processes specific to different cell types are triggered in cells.

For example, macrophages migrate to the area with an increased sodium chloride concentration. On their way, they produce large quantities of vascular endothelial growth factor C (VEGFC), a signaling molecule that promotes angiogenesis and blood flow. This dilutes intercellular fluid and reduces the concentration of ions in the area. Endothelial cells in the hypertensive zone release nitric oxide, a vasodilator that promotes blood flow.

Osmotic mechanisms are also associated with keratinocyte proliferation, maturation, migration, necrosis, and apoptosis. The direction and intensity of these processes depend on the concentration and ionic composition of the medium.

The effect of hypertonic saline solution on the skin mechanoreceptors, which perceive touch and pressure, is realized in the following way. On the plasma membrane of mechanoreceptors, there are Piezo protein channels through which positive ions, including calcium ions, enter the cell (Shin S.M. et al., 2023). The channels open when an external deforming force, either mechanical or intracellular fluid pressure, changes the membrane tension. As a result, mechanoreceptors are activated, which not only transmit a signal to the CNS but also take part in tissue homeostasis regulation at the local level by releasing various mediators.

Concentration, composition, and pH are the main parameters that determine the impact of saline solution on the skin.

The details of the response of different skin cells to the hypertonic solution are still not fully understood. Still, it is known that such a solution is a powerful stimulus to trigger compensatory reactions that generally increase the skin's resistance to various external and internal factors that disturb its homeostasis, mobilizing all protective systems. Of course, these benefits can only be attained if the concentration is not so high as to cause cell death due to osmotic shock.

In addition to concentration, the solution's composition and pH are essential. Different ions and minerals will trigger and control different biochemical reactions, thus ensuring a particular cellular response. It is also critical that the water is not alkaline — its pH should be no more than 7, optimally around 5, i.e., slightly acidified.

Natural thermal and seawater differ in their qualitative composition and the total concentration of dissolved substances, which will induce different skin reactions. Not all springs are recommended for people with skin problems. Some water is safe for drinking but should not be used for bathing. For example, water should have a neutral or slightly alkaline pH for people with gastrointestinal diseases. Still, it should not be used for washing by people with acne, atopic dermatitis, and psoriasis to avoid irritation and disease aggravation.

On the contrary, water from natural springs has a pH of 5.0–5.5, which is beneficial for treating skin diseases. Bathing in it improves skin condition and promotes wound healing. Dissolved organic substances, such as those found in the thermal springs of Avéne and La Roche-Posay in France, impart beneficial properties to natural water.

Therefore, water from each natural source is unique, as are its indications and contraindications. It should be regarded as a medication, and one should avoid self-prescribing and self-treating, instead following the recommendations developed based on years of clinical experience. However, targeted research is necessary to fully unlock each water source's therapeutic potential.

3.2.2. Why Dead Sea water is indicated for the treatment of psoriasis

Dead Sea water contains 345 g of minerals per liter (34.5% or 34.5 g/100 ml). This salt concentration is about 7 to 10 times higher than in ocean water. The relative proportion of NaCl in Dead Sea water is similar to that in the Mediterranean Sea. Still, the content of other salts, such as $MgCl_2$, $CaCl_2$, KCl, and $MgBr_2$, is significantly higher. Interestingly, it is $CaCl_2$ that gives Dead Sea water its oily consistency and leaves a special silky feeling after bathing. Expressed and prolonged moisturization of the *stratum corneum* occurs by the osmotic mechanism described above.

In skin diseases accompanied by a violation of the epidermal barrier, the salt solution reaches the living cells of the epidermis. Bathing in the Dead Sea has a favorable effect, mainly due to its high magnesium content. Magnesium salts bind to water, affect the proliferation and differentiation of epidermal cells, and contribute to restoring the epidermal barrier (Proksch E. et al., 2005).

The biochemical effects of Dead Sea salt therapy have been confirmed *in vitro* and *in vivo*. *In vitro* studies have shown that magnesium bromide and magnesium chloride inhibit the excessive proliferation of keratinocytes characteristic of psoriasis, including by weakening the antigen-presenting ability of Langerhans cells, which are active participants in inflammatory reactions (Katz U. et al., 2012).

3.2.3. Synergism of salt baths and phototherapy

Combining hydrotherapy with Dead Sea salts and phototherapy in natural and artificial conditions is particularly effective.

In a prospective non-randomized study involving 740 patients with psoriasis, complete regression of psoriatic rashes was observed after four weeks of natural balneotherapy and phototherapy at the Dead Sea in 70% of cases (Harari M., Shani J., 1997).

Comparing histologic skin biopsy samples from people with psoriasis before and after undergoing balneotherapy and phototherapy at the Dead Sea, Hodak E. et al. (2003) found a significant decrease in the number of activated T-lymphocytes in the epidermis (by about 90%) and in the dermis (by 77.4% on average).

To understand the individual contribution to the clinical improvements achieved by saltwater bathing and Dead Sea phototherapy, David M. et al. (2000) prospectively compared three treatments: Dead Sea phototherapy alone, Dead Sea water therapy alone, and their combination. These treatment modalities led to 79%, 22.1%, and 87% improvements in PASI scores, respectively, suggesting that phototherapy is the most critical factor. The higher rate of improvement in the combination therapy group can be attributed to the increased skin sensitivity to UV light after exposure to Dead Sea water.

3.2.4. Comparison of natural thalassotherapy at the Dead Sea, salt baths with Dead Sea salts, and conventional salt baths

A meta-analysis comparing the efficacy of artificial thalassotherapy (bathing with Dead Sea salts) combined with phototherapy and natural thalassotherapy and heliotherapy at the Dead Sea was conducted by Katz U. et al. (2012) by analyzing studies published between 1994 and 2014. Both treatments were effective in psoriasis, and their results were comparable.

The results yielded by Halevy S. et al.'s (1997) comparative study of the clinical effect of salt baths with Dead Sea salts and ordinary salts are particularly noteworthy. Their study sample included 25 patients with psoriasis vulgaris with 15% or more of the body surface affected. The participants were randomly divided into two groups and were treated with either Dead Sea salt baths (13 patients) or conventional salt baths (12 patients). The treatment protocol included daily 20-minute salt baths at 35 °C, followed by tap water rinsing and application of white soft paraffin, which was reapplied a few hours later. The treatment was carried out for three weeks. Topical treatment was discontinued two weeks before the start of bathing, and general treatment was discontinued four weeks before the start of bathing. In both groups, the mean PASI value was significantly lower by the end of treatment than before treatment. On the other hand, the mean percentage decrease in PASI score by the end of treatment was higher in the group using Dead Sea salts (34.8% vs. 27.5%). A similar trend was observed one month after discontinuing the treatment protocol (43.6% vs. 24%).

These results indicate that baths with Dead Sea salts and conventional salts have a positive therapeutic effect, similar to monotherapy. However, the positive impact was slightly higher in patients who took baths with Dead Sea salts.

The above findings suggest that salt baths increase skin hydration and have anti-inflammatory and antiproliferative effects. Salt baths can be combined with phototherapy, and emollients with occlusive properties can be applied to the skin after bathing to enhance the clinical impact. This treatment regimen prolongs the effect of increasing skin hydration by creating a film on the skin surface that prevents TEWL.

3.3. Basic skincare products

Basic skincare products are an essential component of a comprehensive psoriasis treatment. They help restore the epidermal barrier, improve skin hydration, and enhance the effects of anti-inflammatory therapy.

Generally, basic skincare should be carried out during exacerbation and remission. It is the basis for successful topical and systemic psoriasis therapy (**Fig. III-3-3**).

Let's look at the skincare products for people with psoriasis.

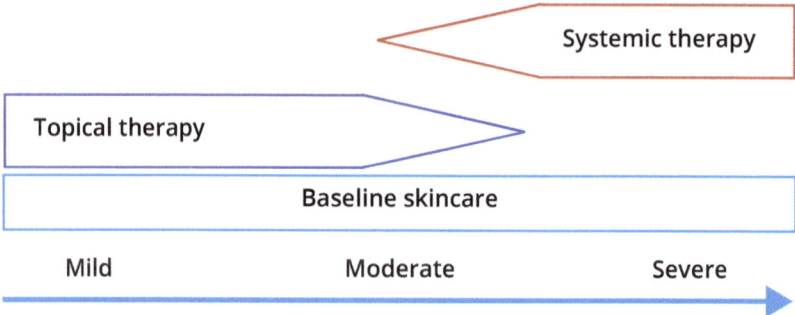

Figure III-3-3. Basic care as a part of an integrated approach to psoriasis treatment (adapted from Luger T. et al., 2014)

3.3.1. Emollients

In psoriasis as well as in atopic dermatitis, emollients play a key role in reducing TEWL, restoring intercellular lipids of the *stratum corneum*, and promoting the formation of a healthy skin microbiome, thus accelerating the restoration of the skin barrier (see Part I, section 3.2). The use of emollients with a mixture of lipids and moisturizers in psoriasis is accompanied by the following effects (Luger T. et al., 2014):

- Increasing the effectiveness and tolerability of primary therapy
- Significant relief of symptoms such as dry skin, itching, burning, and scaling
- Decreased lesion area and PASI value
- Reduced *S. aureus* colonization of the skin
- Increased skin hydration
- Increase in the DLQI

Softening agents include creams, ointments, lotions, bath oils, and soap substitutes. Creams and ointments are preferable to lotions because they have more pronounced occlusive properties. Ointments should be reserved for particularly dry, thickened, or damaged skin and can be used at night. Lighter, less oily creams or lotions are ideal for daytime use in unaffected areas. Individuals affected by psoriasis should use creams, ointments, or lotions frequently and sufficiently to avoid dry skin (Torsekar R., Gautam M.M., 2017).

3.3.2. Urea

Urea is especially effective in skincare for people with psoriasis. Depending on its concentration, urea has different biological effects.

- **Moisturization.** Urea is a low-molecular-weight hygroscopic compound that forms ionic bonds with water molecules; it is a part of NMF and maintains the *stratum corneum*'s hydration level. In the composition of cosmetic products, urea is included as a moisturizing component at concentrations below 10%.
- **Improving transdermal drug delivery.** Urea is also included in drug formulations because it enhances the penetration through

the *stratum corneum* of some therapeutic agents, including topical GCSs (tGCSs). For example, it has been shown that using topical forms of hydrocortisone and triamcinolone acetonide in combination with 10% urea increases the tGCS penetration by 50% (Wohlrab W., 1984).

- **Antiproliferative effect.** According to Grether-Beck S. et al. (2012), at a 10% concentration, urea regulates the expression of genes involved in keratinocyte differentiation and epidermal lipid synthesis (TG-1, involucrin, loricrin, and filaggrin), as well as the production of antimicrobial peptides. *In vitro* and *in vivo* studies show a decrease in DNA synthesis in basal layer cells by about 45% and epidermal thinning by about 20% under the influence of urea (Pan M. et al., 2013).
- **Broad antibacterial activity.** Short-term use of urea-based creams in case of barrier function failure reduces the likelihood of secondary infection.
- **Keratolytic action.** In the stationary/regressive stage of psoriasis involving hyperkeratosis, urea at concentrations exceeding 15% is used as a keratolytic to remove excess horny masses.

Attention! Urea has keratolytic properties, so its long-term use as a skincare product ingredient is questionable due to its disruption of the adhesion of corneocytes to each other and the acceleration of their desquamation. Long-term use of urea on dry, low-sebum skin decreases the density of the spiny layer of the epidermis. In combination with keratolytic action and increased corneocyte desquamation, urea leads to an increase in TEWL.

3.3.3. Hydroxy acids

Alpha-hydroxy acids (AHAs)

AHAs (fruit acids) are water-soluble organic compounds that have found wide application in cosmetology. Glycolic, lactic, almond, malic, tartaric, and citric acids are considered cosmetic ingredients. The intensity of their exfoliating action is determined primarily by the pH of the solution and, to a much lesser extent, by the total AHA concentration.

AHAs exert several significant impacts.

- **Exfoliating.** The shock change of pH gradient in the *stratum corneum* modifies the activity of enzymes responsible for the formation of horny scales and assembly of lipid barrier at the boundary of horny and granular layers, as well as for the desquamation of corneocytes on the surface. The overall enzyme failure will result in "incorrect" horny scales and an altered lipid barrier, and the skin will try to get rid of them as soon as possible to restore the barrier structure.
- **Moisturizing.** Rapid sloughing of corneocytes and epidermis renewal leads to an increase in the content of functionally active NMF in the skin and, consequently, the associated water. Moreover, one of the AHAs, lactic acid, is part of NMF, so it is used primarily to moisturize and loosen the *stratum corneum*.
- **Remodeling.** In response to AHAs, epidermal cells (keratinocytes, free nerve endings, etc.) release various cytokines. These cytokines enter the dermis and stimulate fibroblasts, increasing the synthesis of type I collagen and glycosaminoglycans. Thus, the dermis remodels and thickens.

AHAs can be used in the stationary stage and should be applied locally to the plaque. Creams, lotions, and gels with 5–12% AHA and a pH of 4–5 are recommended for home care. They should be used regularly, and instructions should be strictly followed to achieve visible results. With psoriasis, the maximum effect can be obtained with preparations containing occlusive components, such as petroleum jelly or mineral oil.

In the office, a superficial peel with 20–30% AHA and a pH of 2–3 is allowed.

Polyhydroxy acids (PHAs)

This group includes three substances used in cosmetic dermatology: lactobionic acid, gluconic acid, and gluconolactone.

Due to their dermatological gentleness, PHAs can be used for skin with a weak barrier and increased sensitivity. PHAs help such skin to get rid of horny masses in time, normalize the cell renewal in the epidermis, and strengthen the barrier function.

They exhibit a pronounced moisturizing and unusually mild exfoliating action, which makes them indispensable for caring for pathologically dry skin (ichthyosis, psoriasis).

3.3.4. Salicylic acid

Salicylic acid is a phenol derivative and has a hydroxyl and phenolic group in its molecule. Although this substance is often equated with beta-hydroxy acids (BHAs), its properties and mechanism of action have more similarities with phenol. Unlike AHAs, salicylic acid is poorly soluble in water, so the pH, which determines the effect of AHAs on the skin, is not essential here. Like phenol, salicylic acid breaks the intramolecular stabilizing disulfide bonds of proteins, leading to denaturation of the protein molecule and loss of its original structural and functional properties. Substances acting in this way are called **keratolytics**.

At the epidermis level, any protein structure — including keratin, cornified envelope proteins, desmosomes, proteins of keratinocyte cell membranes, proteolytic enzymes, and enzymes involved in the formation of the lipid barrier — can serve as a target for salicylic acid and other keratolytics. The significant biological effects of salicylic acid include the following:

- **Exfoliating action.** Due to its phenolic group, salicylic acid acts as a keratolytic, denaturing proteins (primarily corneodesmosomes), has a pronounced exfoliating effect, and indirectly stimulates the division of basal keratinocytes.
- **Bactericidal and bacteriostatic action** against Gram-positive and Gram-negative bacteria and fungi (Lebwohl M., 1999).
- **Reduction of skin oiliness.** Since salicylic acid is well soluble in oil, it can penetrate the sebaceous gland and reduce the secretory activity of sebocytes, thus reducing the skin's oiliness.
- **Photoprotection.** Salicylic acid has photoprotective properties at a concentration of ≥1%, but it should not be applied before UVB exposure.

- **Increased bioavailability of other active agents when used in combination.** Salicylic acid is often combined in topical preparations with topical GCSs and calcineurin inhibitors to improve the latter's absorption.

The concentration of salicylic acid in skincare products does not exceed 1%. For peeling, 15–30% salicylic acid is used. The exfoliating effect is directly proportional to the concentration of the preparation and the exposure time.

The main problem of topical application of salicylic acid in psoriasis is the potential risk of chronic or acute systemic intoxication, manifested by burning of the mucosa, headache, symptoms of CNS damage, metabolic acidosis, tinnitus, nausea, and vomiting (Ortonne J. et al., 2009). **Symptoms of intoxication may occur when salicylic acid is applied to a large percentage of the body surface. For this reason, it is inadmissible to use salicylic acid on more than 20% of the body surface area, especially in children under 12 years of age** (Jacobi A. et al., 2015).

A lipid derivative of salicylic acid — lipohydroxy acid (LHA) — can be found in cosmetic products. Due to its lipophilicity and rather high molecular weight, LHA penetrates relatively slowly into the skin, accumulating in the lipid layer of the *stratum corneum* and "loosening" it. This is mainly due to the exfoliating effect of LHA, which is more pronounced than when unmodified salicylic acid is used. LHA acts on corneocytes lying at the depth of 3–4 *stratum corneum* layers. It is at this depth that the enzymatic process of desquamation — the physiological cleavage of protein bridges between horny scales by proteolytic enzymes — begins. Unlike salicylic acid, which acts on any corneodesmosomes, LHA selectively affects only those that have already started to undergo the process of enzymatic destruction. Finally, the nature of corneodesmosome destruction by LHA differs from that of salicylic acid: in the case of LHA, protein bridges are subjected to more severe destruction.

It should be remembered that ointments at 5–10% salicylic acid concentration (as well as ointments containing 20–30% urea) soften the *stratum corneum* but do not remove it. Consequently, softening should be followed by a horny mass removal procedure. During this period, for a few hours after exposure to keratolytic, it is advantageous to take a bath, go to the bath, use a sponge and loofah, and then carefully remove the loose and detached horny masses. Still, it must be remembered that the skin deprived of the *stratum corneum* becomes defenseless and cannot fulfill its barrier function, so overzealousness with any of the above procedures can be harmful. After removing the *stratum corneum*, it is essential to immediately apply the medication, or cream followed by medicines 15–20 minutes later.

3.3.5. Nicotinamide

Nicotinamide (other names — nicotinic acid amide, niacinamide) is a water-soluble form of vitamin B_3. A deficiency of this vitamin causes a condition called pellagra.

Nicotinamide is a classic component of topical agents prescribed for treating psoriasis due to its several positive therapeutic effects (Namazi M.R., 2003):

- **Immunomodulatory action.** It inhibits the production of IL-1, -12, and TNFα, reduces the ability of neutrophils to move to the inflammatory lesion, and prevents the release of histamine from mast cells.
- **Regulation of melanogenesis.** It inhibits melanogenesis by preventing the transfer of melanosomes from melanocytes to keratinocytes.
- **Normalization of microcirculation.** It prevents pathological vasodilation, characteristic of psoriatic plaques, by inhibiting the induction of nitric oxide, a pronounced vasodilator.
- **Restoration of the lipid barrier.** Stimulates ceramide synthesis.
- **Antiproliferative effect.** It has an antiproliferative indirect impact through sphingosine. Sphingosine — one of the main structural elements of sphingolipids that make up cell membranes — is formed by the catabolism of ceramides, is a cell cycle regulator, and reduces basal epidermal cell proliferation.

3.3.6. Birch tar

Birch tar, one of the oldest remedies for psoriasis, is a mixture of aromatic hydrocarbons, resins, phenols, and several other biologically active substances. It is obtained by dry distillation from birch bark. Birch tar has a specific odor and is black with a bluish–greenish or greenish–blue cast.

Birch tar has traditionally been used to treat psoriasis topically. Due to its anti-inflammatory, antiseptic, revitalizing, resolving, and drying properties, it is a popular ingredient in cosmetic care for skin problems.

The positive clinical effects of birch tar application on various dermatoses have not been adequately investigated. However, in recent decades, enough evidence has accumulated to shed light on the mechanisms by which the biological effects of birch tar are realized.

The most beneficial properties of tar in psoriasis skincare are attributed to the presence of aryl hydrocarbon carbazole in its composition (Sekhon S. et al., 2018).

Carbazole is characterized by the following:

- **Anti-inflammatory effect** due to the inhibition of IL-15 and IL-17 and suppression of Th17-lymphocyte activity
- **Antiproliferative action** through activation of the aryl hydrocarbon receptor (AhR), which is responsible for normal keratinocyte differentiation
- **Inhibition of pathologic angiogenesis**

Thus, due to its active components, birch tar affects different links in the pathogenesis of psoriasis. This ensures that this natural ingredient remains one of the most widely used components of local medical and cosmetic products for psoriasis.

3.4. Peculiarities of basic care and choice of aesthetic treatment depending on the stage of the disease

When selecting skincare products and aesthetic treatments, the stage of the disease should be considered. Emollients can be regarded as the foundation of basic care at any stage of psoriasis.

3.4.1. Progressive stage

The acute stage of psoriasis is characterized by the positive Koebner phenomenon — the appearance of fresh rashes in the irritation area, including mechanical, chemical, or thermal damage. For this reason, aggressive traumatizing agents and procedures should be avoided as much as possible.

At-home care for affected and healthy skin should exclude alcohol-containing products, scrubs, gommage, retinoids (retinoic acid, retinol, tazarotene, adapalene), and AHAs.

Professional procedures such as exfoliation, chemical peels, intense and/or prolonged massage, vaporization, hygienic cleansing, warming masks, injectables, abrasive and laser treatments, microneedling, surgical interventions, and waxing are not allowed.

3.4.2. Stationary/regressive stage

At these stages of the disease, psoriasis lesions are characterized by pronounced hyperkeratosis. Professional care can be extended to treat it — exfoliation, superficial peels, intensive and prolonged massage, vaporization, hygienic cleansing, and masks are allowed.

Peels can also be selectively applied to skin lesion areas. Subsequently, superficial acid and keratolytic peels are preferred. The use of PHA has also shown promising results.

Enzyme peels should not be used. In psoriatic skin, the activity of the proteolytic enzymes of the *stratum corneum* is increased even at the clinical well-being stage. Applying more proteolytic enzymes to the skin may exacerbate the disease.

Injectable carboxytherapy is possible for localized treatment of long-standing psoriatic plaques. It consists of an intradermal injection of CO_2 using a 30 G needle, a 15–30° puncture angle, and a 5 ml/min flow. The injections are performed 2 cm apart. The recommended number of sessions is 5–15, which should be performed twice weekly.

In general, procedures that do not damage the skin are permissible. However, photo and laser hair removal should be avoided during retinoid treatment and for a month after completion.

3.5. Nail care

One of the manifestations of psoriasis, along with rashes on the trunk and scalp, are nail lesions — psoriatic onychopathy. In rare cases, nail psoriasis may be the only symptom of dermatosis (Schons K.R. et al., 2015). The most characteristic pathological changes of the nail plate are:

- Numerous dimple-shaped depressions (**Fig. III-3-4**)
- Discoloration
- Subungual hyperkeratosis
- Onycholysis (separation of the nail plate from the nail bed, **Fig. III-3-5**)
- Yellow and oily nail plates (**Fig. III-3-6**)

These changes are challenging to treat and, in some cases, remain in remission. The unaesthetic appearance of nails affected by psoriasis reduces patients' quality of life and prompts them to seek solutions to aesthetic problems from aestheticians, podologists, manicurists, and pedicurists.

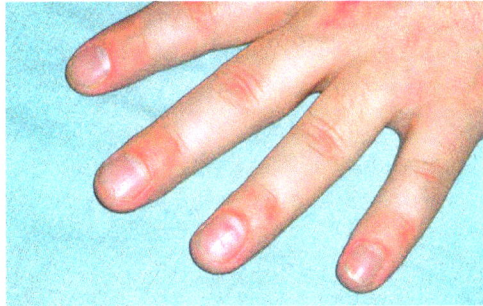

Figure III-3-4. Thimble-shaped depressions (photo provided by V.I. Albanova)

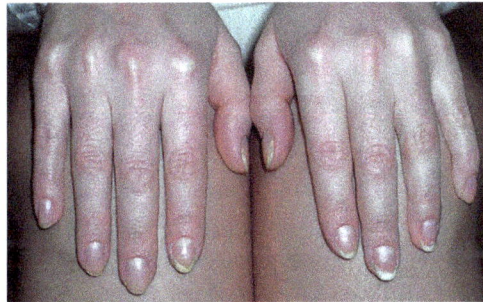

Figure III-3-5. Subnail hyperkeratosis and onycholysis (photo provided by V.I. Albanova)

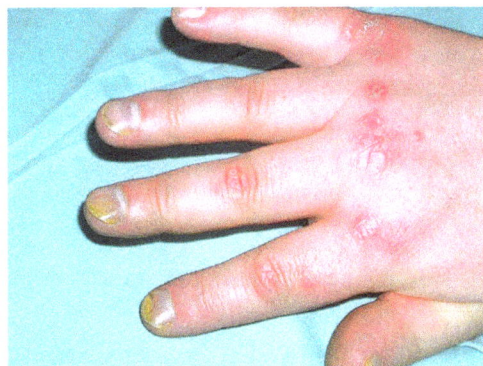

Figure III-3-6. Oily nail plates (photo provided by V.I. Albanova)

In the acute stage of the disease, trauma to the nails and fingers must be avoided. Manicures, trimming, and cleaning the subungual spaces can provoke the Koebner phenomenon. For this reason, nail care should be delicate. Short nail trimming, cuticle preservation, and minimal file use are recommended.

Exposure to chemicals can worsen the existing onychopathy. When performing cosmetic camouflage, it is better to use gel or shellac. A single gel layer is recommended to reduce the UV dose and facilitate its subsequent removal. During the procedure, it is necessary to protect the skin of fingers and hands from UV radiation.

Methods recommended for psoriasis:
- **Biogel.** A soft hypoallergenic material, often enriched with vitamins and minerals, is used to restore and strengthen the nail while providing a natural look.
- **Silicone or polyurethane overlays.** Custom-made overlays adhere to the nail using special glue, providing a protective barrier and improving aesthetics. These materials are flexible, non-allergenic, and ensure gentle adhesion.
- **Polymer-based prosthetics (during remission).** Elastic and durable polymer materials are used to restore missing parts of the nail. They are suitable for psoriasis if hypoallergenic materials are employed and an experienced technician performs the procedure.
- **Gel prosthetics (with caution and hypoallergenic materials).** Special gel materials create a thin layer that mimics a natural nail. The gel is applied in layers and cured under a UV or LED lamp. It is suitable for psoriasis only during remission and without significant inflammation. The gel must be hypoallergenic.

These techniques help reduce or completely relieve pressure on the nail fold, reduce pain and inflammation, and allow for gradual correction of abnormal nail and nail bed growth. However, these manipulations must be avoided in the presence of acute inflammation in the treated area, infectious processes, complete nail absence, or trauma to the nail bed.

NOT recommended for psoriasis:

- **Acrylic prosthetics (due to harsh chemicals).** Acrylic powder is mixed with a monomer to form a malleable substance shaped into an artificial nail. Once hardened, it is polished to achieve the desired appearance. Acrylic materials can irritate the skin and worsen the condition.
- **Techniques involving trauma to the nail plate (e.g., fiberglass and resin).** Fiberglass is applied to a damaged nail area and secured with resin for strength and support. However, this technique is unsuitable for psoriasis, as a resin may cause allergies and irritation and can traumatize the nail plate.
- **Laser interventions if the condition is active.** A laser removes damaged nail tissue and models a new artificial layer using biocompatible materials. It can be used for psoriasis cautiously, as the laser can irritate the skin and exacerbate inflammation.

Important: A dermatologist and a nail prosthetics specialist must always be consulted before selecting a nail treatment method.

3.6. Hair care

In adult patients, the scalp is often the first site of lesion formation and remains involved to a greater or lesser extent for many years. At the same time, lesions that subsequently appear elsewhere may go into remission.

Many patients develop scalp lesions in their first years, often in infancy. Some children are diagnosed with gneiss, a marker of psoriasis. Typical psoriatic plaques have well-defined borders and thick gray–white scales. They can appear in the presence or absence of other forms of psoriasis.

The severity of psoriasis varies, ranging from slight desquamation and erythema with minimal tissue thickening to the appearance of markedly inflamed and crusted plaque-like lesions and even asbestos rash with the formation of pronounced scabs covering the proximal parts of the hair fibers. The pathological process often involves areas adjacent to the scalp (forehead, temples, ears, and occiput), where lesions may transfer from the scalp or develop independently (**Fig. III-3-7**) (Phiske M.M., 2016).

Three degrees of severity of scalp psoriasis are described:

1. **Mild** — areas of dry, flaky skin on the scalp, interspersed with patches of healthy skin. The hairline is not involved in the pathological process, and there is no hair loss.

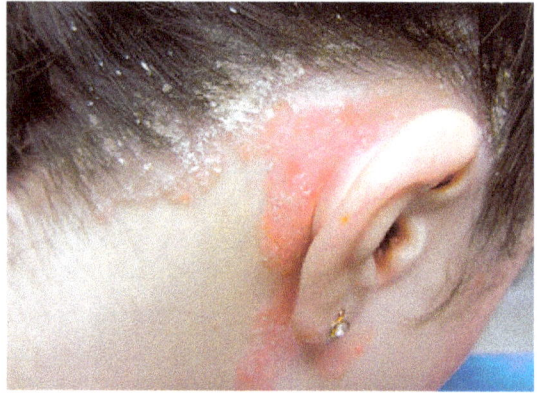

Figure III-3-7. Lesions on the scalp and behind the ear (photo provided by V.I. Albanova)

2. **Moderate** — areas of dry, flaky skin and scales covering a more significant portion of the scalp, with small gaps of normal skin. Lesions extend to the hairline, with minimal hair loss noted.

3. **Severe** — lesions spread across the entire scalp, with only a minimal amount of normal skin remaining. Thick, nodular scales are present. The hairline is affected, and areas of lesions with erythema and scales extend beyond it. Temporary hair loss may occur.

The rashes are often accompanied by itching. Scratching the lesions and attempting to remove crusts and scales can result in wetting, increased itching, and further lesion growth. The patient should be warned against touching the hair, combing, and rubbing the skin with hands or a brush.

The Asia Scalp Psoriasis Study Group (ASPSG) advocates for a patient-centered approach, as it facilitates treatment-related decisions that consider both the objective and subjective severity of scalp psoriasis at an individual level. Treating physicians should consider aspects such as the patient's quality of life, the initial response to therapy, preference for different drug release forms, patient compliance (treatment adherence), cost of the therapeutic course, availability of free time for treatments, patient's capacity for self-monitoring, and possible adverse events.

Previously utilized treatments included cutting off superficial skin layers, phototherapy, pulsating magnetic fields, and Grenz rays. One of the first topical agents developed for this patient group was a mixture of liquid petroleum jelly, sodium chloride solution, and phenol.

The current approach involves first-line topical agents (**Table III-3-1**), where treatment choice should be guided by disease severity, patient preference, previous response to therapy, and cost. The active ingredients in the formulations and those that form the basis of the drugs influence efficacy, tolerability, and treatment adherence.

Table III-3-1. Means and methods of psoriasis treatment

FIRST-LINE THERAPY	SECOND-LINE THERAPY
• Topical corticosteroids • Vitamin D3 analogs (calcipotriol) • Salicylic acid/urea • Ditranol/antralin • Coal tar • Tazarotene	• Phototherapy • Systemic therapy (methotrexate, acitretin, cyclosporine) • Biologicals

The drug can be washed off (shampoo) or applied to the scalp (alcohol-containing lotion, gel, foam, cream, ointment, oil).

Active ingredients include keratolytic compounds, coal tar, ditranol, retinoids, antifungal agents, corticosteroids, and vitamin D_3 analogs (**Table III-3-2**).

Treatment of scalp psoriasis is divided into four stages:

1. **Cleansing** with salicylic acid or urea preparations to remove scales
2. **Reducing inflammation and healing** by tGCSs, vitamin D analogs, tar, dithranol, antifungal agents, UV light, or systemic medications
3. **Stabilization** with administration of a steroid-sparing analog on weekdays and a highly active topical corticosteroid on weekends
4. **Maintaining remission** by using a vitamin D analog as monotherapy or in conjunction with tar shampoo

Table III-3-2. Topical therapy for scalp psoriasis (Phiske M.M., 2016)

TOPICAL PREPARATIONS	DESCRIPTION
Topical steroids	• Helpful for localized lesions but require physician monitoring
Vitamin D analogs	• Pleasant to use • Contraindicated in pregnancy and during breastfeeding • May be used in combination with corticosteroid ointments for a short time
Keratolytics	• Help reduce excessive scaling, but may irritate skin adjacent to lesions
Ditranol (including short contact therapy)	• Good for treating chronic plaque psoriasis in specific areas
Vitamin A analogs	• Applied once a day • Not recommended for use on the face, skinfolds, or large areas of the body • Contraindicated in pregnancy and during breastfeeding
Tar preparations	• Help remove loose scales • Leave dirty residue and stain clothes
Emollients (moisturizers)	• Relieve itching, reduce skin dryness and scaling, soften cracks, and promote penetration of other topical agents • A 10% urea solution and a 10% lactic acid solution are often used as scalp moisturizers

Keratolytic agents, prescribed as ointments and creams, do not wash off well from hair, leaving it looking unkempt. Therefore, for very oily hair, it is better to apply them in the evening and wash them off with shampoo in the morning. After washing, conditioners should also be used to detach the scales stuck to the hair shaft.

If the lesions are mild, it is preferable to use therapeutic shampoos containing tar, salicylic acid, or zinc, along with special conditioner-balm rinses. Hair masks with anti-inflammatory ingredients are also beneficial. At least once a week, 1–2 hours before washing, vegetable oil (burdock, olive, or coconut) is massaged into the affected areas, followed by wearing a plastic cap and wrapping the head with a towel. Itching and inflammation are reduced by rinsing the hair with herbal decoctions — nettle, oak bark, sage, lavender, and mint.

After washing, the hair is dried with a hair dryer, holding it at a 15 cm distance from the head while maintaining a constant airflow (warm, but not hot). It is better to comb dry hair, which should be done slowly and carefully to avoid damaging the affected skin. Electric hair pluckers, electric styling brushes, curling irons, flat irons, and thermal rollers are undesirable for hair styling. It is better to avoid complex styling, lacquer, and many styling products and tightening the hair with an elastic band. In the progressive stage, perm and hair coloring are contraindicated. Generally, it is easier to care for short hair, so a beautiful haircut can be a good solution.

Chapter 4
Nutrition and nutraceutical support

Because psoriasis is a chronic inflammatory disease that can be controlled but not cured, many patients seek to improve their condition and alleviate symptoms through alternative methods and lifestyle changes. The disease and the approaches offered are so variable that it is difficult to assess the contribution of any individual lifestyle component. A review of available publications indicates dietary modifications have the most beneficial effect on the psoriasis course. Most diets have a mixed impact on disease manifestations, although some individual foods are helpful. Foods and supplements with systemic anti-inflammatory effects appear more likely to improve psoriasis symptoms.

In a 2017 survey of 1,206 people with psoriasis, 86% of respondents reported changing their diet due to the disease (Afifi L. et al., 2017). In addition, when comparing the dietary preferences of people with psoriasis and healthy participants of the same gender and similar age, it was shown that people with psoriasis ate significantly less sugar, whole-grain fiber, dairy products, and calcium. The survey also revealed that patients' diets contained considerably more fruits, vegetables, and legumes. Although patients did not follow a single diet, 40% reported trying a specialized diet to correct psoriasis. Mediterranean and vegetarian diets were most strongly associated with alleviation of psoriasis symptoms. Finally, specific dietary components were reported more frequently to lead to improvement in psoriasis symptoms, particularly increased consumption of fish oil, fruits, vegetables, and water. Reducing alcohol, gluten, nightshade, and junk food intake was associated with improved skin condition in at least 50% of patients.

4.1. The Mediterranean diet

The Mediterranean diet includes many fruits, vegetables, nuts and legumes, cereals, and olive oil. However, red meat, dairy products, and alcohol (except red wine) are limited (**Fig. III-4-1**).

The diet as a whole, rather than individual components, is likely to yield good results. The various elements work together to reduce inflammation and have a beneficial effect on the body.

Some key aspects of the Mediterranean diet are:

- Relatively high fat intake (30–50% of total daily calories) mainly due to monounsaturated fatty acids (olive oil); saturated fat accounts for less than 8% of calories

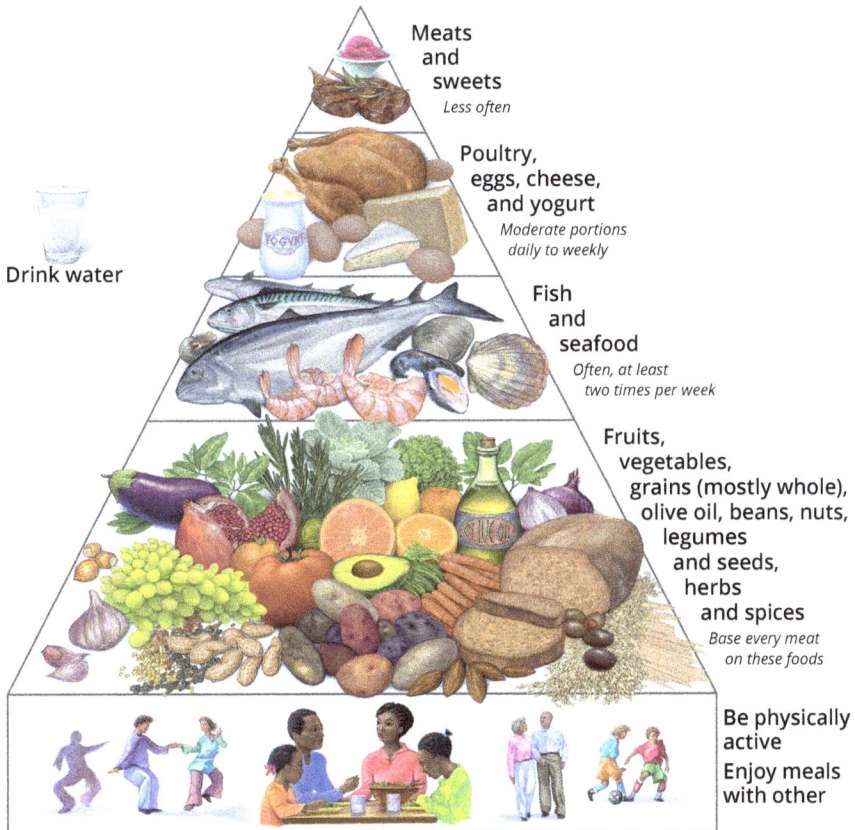

Meats and sweets
Less often

Poultry, eggs, cheese, and yogurt
Moderate portions daily to weekly

Drink water

Fish and seafood
Often, at least two times per week

Fruits, vegetables, grains (mostly whole), olive oil, beans, nuts, legumes and seeds, herbs and spices
Base every meat on these foods

Be physically active
Enjoy meals with other

Figure III-4-1. Mediterranean diet is most strongly associated with the alleviation of psoriasis symptoms

- High intake of omega-3 fatty acids from fish (two or more servings per week) and plant sources
- A low ratio of omega-6 to omega-3 fatty acids, approximately 2–3:1 compared to the 14:1 ratio typical of the U.S. and European diets
- Consumption of fruits and vegetables in large quantities
- High fiber intake (32 g/day)
- Low amounts of simple and rapidly digestible carbohydrates (i.e., low glycemic load)

Adherence to this dietary protocol is associated with a reduced risk of cardiovascular disease, rheumatoid arthritis, and Crohn's disease, possibly due to the inclusion of a large number and variety of foods containing antioxidants and anti-inflammatory compounds, including monounsaturated fatty acids (MUFAs) in olive oil and polyphenols in fruits and vegetables. Consumption of PUFAs and nutrients with potent anti-inflammatory properties is associated with a reduced risk of developing chronic inflammatory diseases. Levels of PUFA intake have been reported to be a prognostic factor for psoriasis severity: patients with severe psoriasis are characterized by low dietary PUFA intake.

Authors of several studies have attempted to quantify the association between the Mediterranean diet and psoriasis. For instance, as a part of their cross-sectional study involving 62 people with psoriasis, Barrea L. et al. (2015) examined the relationship between dermatosis severity and adherence to the Mediterranean diet using a 14-item questionnaire. Their results showed that patients with severe psoriasis and high C-reactive protein levels had lower adherence to the diet. Notably, the level of extra virgin olive oil consumption was inversely correlated with psoriasis severity, and the level of fish consumption was associated with the level of C-reactive protein, a marker of inflammation.

In another study involving 3,557 patients surveyed using a cross-sectional questionnaire, Phan C. et al. (2018) established a similar relationship: patients with severe psoriasis reported low adherence to the Mediterranean diet.

Although a causal relationship between diet and psoriasis severity is yet to be examined, several authors have reported potential effects of pro-inflammatory and anti-inflammatory dietary components on disease severity.

Common foods and nutrients that exhibit anti-inflammatory properties include PUFAs, fish, vitamins A, C, D, and E, and omega-3 fatty acids. Because many factors can influence the findings of dietary studies based on questionnaires, it is difficult to state that the Mediterranean diet is unequivocally beneficial for psoriasis. Nevertheless, certain diet components can predict psoriasis severity, and this diet can be combined with other treatments.

4.2. Anti-inflammatory diet

Numerous studies of the relationship between dietary patterns and chronic disease have contributed to developing an anti-inflammatory diet, which corrects or halts the inflammatory process. In basic terms, the anti-inflammatory diet is like the Mediterranean diet. It can be recommended to people with psoriasis as another mechanism to influence the course of the disease.

The basics of an anti-inflammatory diet are summarized below.

4.2.1. Increased proportion of foods with anti-inflammatory properties in the diet

Brightly colored fruits and vegetables

Brightly colored fruits and vegetables, mainly green, orange, yellow, red, and purple, contain important antioxidants and are characterized by powerful anti-inflammatory effects.

Fruit and vegetable intake should be maximized. The quantity of legumes (beans and peas) and fruits and vegetables — including dark green, orange, yellow, red, and purple — should be equivalent to at least 4.5 cups daily. For light "airy" vegetables, such as lettuce and raw spinach, one "head" is considered equal to 0.5 cup. Red berries, as well as vegetables in the Cruciferous family — broccoli (*Brassica silvestris*), napa cabbage (*Brassica rapa*), wild cabbage (*Brassica oleracea*), and cauliflower (*Brassicaoleracea var. botrytis*) — are particularly rich in anti-inflammatory compounds.

The amount of foods from each food group with the same nutritional value is determined using a cup equivalent. Vegetables: 1 cup equivalent of vegetables equals 1 cup of raw vegetables (or vegetable juice) or 2 cups of leafy salad greens. Fruits: 1 cup equivalent equals 1 cup of fruits or 0.5 cup of fruit juice.

Vegetable oils

Vegetable oils are extracted from raw plant materials (fruits, seeds, pips) and consist of triglycerides of fatty acids and associated substances (phospholipids, free fatty acids, waxes, sterols, coloring substances, etc.). To produce vegetable oils, press and extraction methods and their combinations are used (double pressing and pressing followed by extraction). Vegetable oils obtained by pressing or extraction contain associated substances that determine their quality. To get oil with a good marketable appearance, remove hazardous substances, and increase shelf life, oils are subjected to purification using various refining methods. The degree of purification directly affects the beneficial properties of the oil.

Natural (virgin) means that the oil has been obtained using only physical methods without chemical purification. Refined means the oil has been refined using physical and chemical processes to remove strong flavor (usually unwanted) and acid content (free fatty acids). In general, refined oil is considered less healthy than natural oil.

Olive oil contains mostly monounsaturated fatty acids (not omega-3 or -6). It helps reduce blood pressure, LDL cholesterol, and signs of inflammation. According to the International Olive Council's standards, varieties made only from natural oil — labeled Extra-virgin olive oil (EVOO) and Virgin olive oil — are the healthiest. Oils labeled Pure olive oil or Olive oil are usually a blend of purified and natural oil. Olive-pomace oil is a purified cake oil extracted from the pressings using chemical solvents, usually hexane, and subjected to heat-based treatments. It is sometimes blended with natural oil. This type of oil is quite suitable for food, but it cannot be called proper olive oil.

Pure olive oil and Virgin olive oil are best suited for cooking. On the contrary, EVOO should not be used for cooking, as heating it even to a moderate temperature will reduce its beneficial properties. This type of oil is best added after cooking or used as a salad dressing.

Canola oil is a good option primarily because it contains monoun-saturated fatty acids but lacks many beneficial characteristics of olive oil. Other oils with moderate concentrations of monounsaturated fatty acids, such as **peanut**, **sesame**, and **rice bran**, also contain moderate amounts of omega-6 fatty acids.

Oils such as **soybean**, **corn**, **sunflower**, **safflower**, **grapeseed**, **cottonseed**, **wheat germ**, and foods prepared with them are high in omega-6 fatty acids. Psoriasis patients should reduce their amount in diet. They should favor sources of monounsaturated fatty acids, such as olive and canola oils, and increase the intake of foods rich in ome-ga-3 (e.g., fatty cold-water fish). The vegetable seed oils listed above are not unhealthy in limited amounts but tend to be consumed in ex-cessive quantities as a part of the Western diet.

The impact of omega-6 fatty acids on inflammation and chronic dis-ease remains unclear. Early studies showed that high levels of these dietary fatty acids are associated with pro-inflammatory pathways in the body. However, recent work suggests that omega-6 fatty acids may not directly increase inflammation. In some cases, they can exert anti-inflammatory effects depending on other factors. However, it is clear that omega-3 fatty acids have anti-inflammatory effects, hence their considerable health benefits. Since vegetable oils are often used for cooking, limiting the consumption of heat-treated foods is the best way to reduce omega-6 intake.

Omega-3 fatty acids

Foods containing long-chain omega-3 fatty acids, such as cold-wa-ter fish (salmon, sardines, and tuna), are particularly helpful in reduc-ing inflammation. Psoriasis patients should aim for 2–3 servings per week (a serving is approximately 70 g) of oily fish (salmon, mackerel, herring, lake trout, sardines, and longfin tuna). Fish oil is rich in ome-ga-3 fatty acids such as eicosapentaenoic acid (EPA) and docosahexae-noic acid (DHA), which are more potent anti-inflammatory agents than α-linolenic acid (ALA), commonly found in plants. ALA is converted to EPA and then to DHA, but less than 1% of the original amount of ALA is converted to physiologically active EPA and DHA. For this reason, flaxseed oil, rich in ALA, is not as effective as EPA and DHA in combat-ting inflammation.

Although vegan supplements derived from algae contain both EPA and DHA, it is better to supplement the diet with high-quality fish oil (1 g of fish oil contains about 0.5–1 g of combined omega-3 fatty acids, so 3–4 g is the correct daily amount). In chronic inflammatory conditions, the amount can be increased to 4–5 g daily.

Green tea, turmeric, ginger
These foods contain many critical anti-inflammatory components and should be included in the diet. For example, they can be used to prepare tea or as spices in cooking.

Products containing magnesium
Magnesium (Mg) deficiency is associated with increased inflammation. Dark green leafy vegetables, legumes, nuts, seeds, and whole grains are rich sources of Mg. The recommended dietary intake of Mg is 320 and 420 mg/d for women and men over 31, respectively. Exceeding this amount does not provide additional beneficial effects. One cup of spinach or mangold contains about 150 mg, 0.5 cup of pumpkin seeds contains 190 mg, and 1 cup of black beans, 3/4 cup of quinoa, and 1/4 cup of cashews or sunflower seeds contain about 120 mg.

Vitamin D
Most people have vitamin D insufficiency or deficiency, which is a significant issue in psoriasis as it affects the severity of the disease (see Part II, section 4.3). Daily intake of vitamin D-rich foods is a simple and inexpensive alternative to treatment.

The best sources of vitamin D_3 are cod liver (canned), fatty fish (salmon, trout, herring, mackerel), and, to a much lesser extent, egg yolks and animal liver. Some plant products can also be sources of vitamin D_2: edible mushrooms, such as maitake, portobello, and chanterelles.

Vitamin D absorption occurs in the duodenum and small intestine in the presence of bile acids. In the gastrointestinal tract, vitamin D is incorporated into micelles formed by bile acids and enters enterocytes. It enters the bloodstream with chylomicrons through lymphatic vessels, where it is further metabolized in the same way as vitamin D formed in the skin. However, even foods high in vitamin D do not satisfy the body's requirements. Due to insufficient vitamin D intake from food, guidelines are developed for oral vitamin D supplementation (Holick M.F. et al., 2011; Mattozzi C. et al., 2016).

Nutritional supplements and vitamins (lozenges, tablets, capsules, solutions, juices, fruit purees, etc.) with different vitamin D content are sold in pharmacies and online. They are intended to prevent vitamin D deficiency but can also be used for treatment.

The doctor prescribes medications based on the vitamin D blood test results. A maintenance dose is required once the optimal vitamin D content has been reached. Nutritional supplements may also be used during this period. Prophylactic doses may be prescribed without prior laboratory testing.

4.2.2. Reducing blood sugar levels

Limiting the proportion of refined carbohydrates in the diet

Foods high in refined carbohydrates, such as white flour, white rice, white bread, and refined sugar, are quickly broken down by the body into simple sugars. As they are rapidly absorbed, they can cause significant spikes in insulin, a hormone with pro-inflammatory properties. It is best to limit or avoid these foods.

Foods with a low glycemic index

Low-glycemic-index foods like whole grains, starch-containing vegetables, and fruits are recommended. These fiber-rich foods, which include complex carbohydrates, help maintain stable blood sugar levels and reduce insulin's pro-inflammatory effects. Eating complex carbohydrates and foods high in dietary fiber and healthy oils slows the breakdown of carbohydrates and reduces the overall glycemic load.

Inclusion in the diet of a large number of foods high in dietary fiber

Dietary fiber slows the absorption of carbohydrates, helps regulate blood sugar levels, and prolongs the feeling of satiety after a meal.

The mechanisms by which dietary fiber reduces inflammation are not well understood. Nonetheless, it is well known that dietary fiber promotes the processing of fats in the body and creates favorable conditions for a healthy gut microbiome with immunomodulatory and anti-inflammatory activity. Natural foods rich in dietary fiber contain other essential anti-inflammatory nutrients. The optimal nutritional intake is at least 30 g of dietary fiber daily.

4.2.3. Reduced intake of foods with pro-inflammatory properties

Trans fats
Trans fats (fatty acid trans-isomers, "hydrogenated oils") are unsaturated fats that contribute to inflammation. Trans fats are found in margarine, deep-fried foods, and processed foods designed to last a long time, such as crackers and snacks.

Dairy products
High-fat and unfermented dairy products may slightly increase inflammation. In contrast, fermented dairy products such as yogurt and kefir positively affect the course of inflammatory diseases and reduce the risk of cardiovascular disorders. Therefore, consuming moderate amounts of fermented dairy products, especially yogurt, may be an acceptable part of anti-inflammatory nutrition.

Red meat
Large amounts of red meat in the diet — especially ready-to-eat meat products such as hot dogs, sausages, and frankfurters — are associated with a high risk of cardiovascular disease and cancer. Although red meat is a source of protein, iron, and other micronutrients, poultry, eggs, dairy products, plant proteins (legumes), and grains may serve as adequate substitutes. When consuming red meat, preference should be given to lean varieties, and any visible fat should be removed. The World Cancer Research Fund suggests consuming no more than 350–500 g of cooked red meat weekly. Foods such as ham, salami, hot dogs, and sausages should be avoided.

Fried food

Consuming foods with a toasted crust stimulates inflammatory responses.

The effect of the anti-inflammatory diet takes some time to manifest; hence, clinical improvement will be noticeable after about six weeks. An anti-inflammatory diet should be part of a broader strategy to maintain long-term health.

Sufficient physical activity, normalization of sleep, and stress avoidance can be considered additional recommendations for controlling chronic inflammation. Together with an anti-inflammatory diet, these practices form the basis of an "anti-inflammatory" lifestyle (**Fig. III-4-2**).

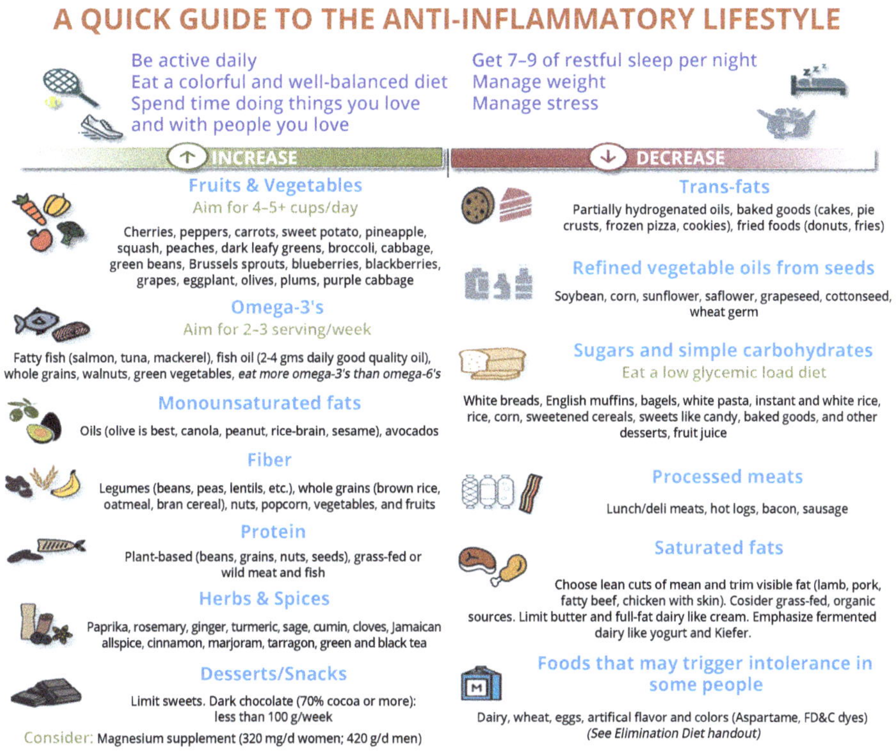

A QUICK GUIDE TO THE ANTI-INFLAMMATORY LIFESTYLE

Be active daily
Eat a colorful and well-balanced diet
Spend time doing things you love and with people you love

Get 7–9 of restful sleep per night
Manage weight
Manage stress

↑ INCREASE

Fruits & Vegetables
Aim for 4–5+ cups/day

Cherries, peppers, carrots, sweet potato, pineapple, squash, peaches, dark leafy greens, broccoli, cabbage, green beans, Brussels sprouts, blueberries, blackberries, grapes, eggplant, olives, plums, purple cabbage

Omega-3's
Aim for 2–3 serving/week

Fatty fish (salmon, tuna, mackerel), fish oil (2-4 gms daily good quality oil), whole grains, walnuts, green vegetables, *eat more omega-3's than omega-6's*

Monounsaturated fats

Oils (olive is best, canola, peanut, rice-brain, sesame), avocados

Fiber

Legumes (beans, peas, lentils, etc.), whole grains (brown rice, oatmeal, bran cereal), nuts, popcorn, vegetables, and fruits

Protein

Plant-based (beans, grains, nuts, seeds), grass-fed or wild meat and fish

Herbs & Spices

Paprika, rosemary, ginger, turmeric, sage, cumin, cloves, Jamaican allspice, cinnamon, marjoram, tarragon, green and black tea

Desserts/Snacks

Limit sweets. Dark chocolate (70% cocoa or more): less than 100 g/week

Consider: Magnesium supplement (320 mg/d women; 420 g/d men)

↓ DECREASE

Trans-fats

Partially hydrogenated oils, baked goods (cakes, pie crusts, frozen pizza, cookies), fried foods (donuts, fries)

Refined vegetable oils from seeds

Soybean, corn, sunflower, saflower, grapeseed, cottonseed, wheat germ

Sugars and simple carbohydrates
Eat a low glycemic load diet

White breads, English muffins, bagels, white pasta, instant and white rice, rice, corn, sweetened cereals, sweets like candy, baked goods, and other desserts, fruit juice

Processed meats

Lunch/deli meats, hot logs, bacon, sausage

Saturated fats

Choose lean cuts of mean and trim visible fat (lamb, pork, fatty beef, chicken with skin). Cosider grass-fed, organic sources. Limit butter and full-fat dairy like cream. Emphasize fermented dairy like yogurt and Kiefer.

Foods that may trigger intolerance in some people

Dairy, wheat, eggs, artifical flavor and colors (Aspartame, FD&C dyes)
(See Elimination Diet handout)

Figure III-4-2. The Anti-Inflammatory Lifestyle Patient Handout, University of Wisconsin Integrative Health

4.3. Probiotics

Probiotics improve the course of psoriasis through the development of a healthy gut microbiome. Examples of some of the mechanisms by which probiotics may influence the gut microbiome include:

- Decrease in pH, creating a more acidic microenvironment unfavorable to pathogenic microorganisms
- Competition with unwanted microorganisms for nutrition
- Production of strain-specific antimicrobial compounds such as bacteriocins
- Restoring the population of health-benefiting bacteria
- Reduction of harmful bacterial metabolites
- Absorption and breakdown of carbohydrates
- Production of vitamins (vitamin B and vitamin K), antioxidants, polyphenols, and conjugated linoleic acid
- Immune system development at an early age
- Support for a healthy immune system throughout life
- Maintenance of intestinal barrier function
- Molecular signaling to distant organs by activating receptors on neurons present in the digestive tract

Fermented milk bacteria (*Bifidobacterium* and *Lactobacillus*) have the most valuable biological effects (Yamashiro Y., 2022).

Lactobacillus and *Bifidobacteria* produce numerous bactericidal substances such as lactic acid, bacteriocins, bacteriocin-like substances, and short-chain fatty acids (SCFAs) (Kierasińska M., Donskow-Łysoniewska K., 2021). SCFAs are involved in communication between the gut microbiome and the immune system. They reduce the risk of inflammation by inhibiting histone deacetylase, which leads to increased acetylation of histone H3 in the promoter region of the FOXP3 gene, characteristic of Treg-lymphocytes, and activation of Treg*.

---

* T regulatory T cells (Treg) are central regulators of the immune response. Their primary function is to control the strength and duration of the immune response by regulating the function of T effector cells (T-helper cells and T-killers). These T-lymphocytes express FOXP3, a transcription factor that regulates the transcription of genes responsible for T cell differentiation and the expression of cytokines and other factors involved in suppressing the immune response.

Table III-4-1 summarizes the current data on using probiotics to modulate skin homeostasis and treat psoriasis.

Table III-4-1. Overview of clinical studies on the use of probiotics in psoriasis

STUDY	PROBIOTIC STRAIN	RESULTS
One patient with pustular psoriasis, 6 months (Vijayashankar M., Raghunath N., 2012)	*Lactobacillus sporogenes*	Regression of rashes by two weeks and complete disappearance by six months was observed
27 patients with psoriasis, 12 weeks (Lin C. et al., 2021)	*Bacteroides fragillis*	Significant decrease in the PASI value
50 patients with plaque psoriasis, 8 weeks (Moludi J. et al., 2021)	Probiotic blend: *Lactobacillus acidophilus, Bifidobacterium spp. bifidum, B. lactis, B. langum*	• Decrease in Beck Depression Index (BDI) and DLQI • Decrease in PASI and Psoriasis Symptom Scale scores • Increase in total anti-oxidant capacity • Decrease in C-reactive protein and IL-6 levels
64 patients with mild to moderate psoriasis severity, 12 weeks (Akbarzadeh A. et al., 2022)	Capsules containing 7 probiotic strains (*Lactobacillus casei, L. acidophilus, L. rhamnosus, L. bulgaricus, Bifidobacterium breve, B. longum, Streptococcus thermophiles*) and a prebiotic	Increased serum levels of Fe, Zn, P, Mg, Ca, and Na in the group of patients taking probiotics, indicating better mineral absorption
90 patients with plaque psoriasis, 12 weeks (Navarro-López V. et al., 2019)	Probiotic blend: *Bifidobacterium longum* CECT 7347, *B. lactis* CECT 8145, *Lactobacillus rhamnosus* CECT 8361	Significant reduction in PASI score and recurrence rate

Continued on p. 230

STUDY	PROBIOTIC STRAIN	RESULTS
27 patients with psoriasis, 6–8 weeks (Groeger D. et al., 2013)	*Bifidobacteria*	Decrease in plasma levels of C-reactive protein and TNFα
45 patients with psoriasis, 8 weeks (Siu P.L.K. et al., 2024)	Probiotic blend: *Lactobacillus plantarum* GKM3, *L. brevis* GKL9, *L. acidophilus* GKA7, *L. casei* GKC1, *L. reuteri* GKR1, *L. gasseri* GKG1, *Bifidobacterium bifidum* GKB2, *B. longum* GKL7	• Regression of comorbidities, including irritable bowel syndrome, functional constipation, and functional diarrhea • Increase in the DLQI scores • Reduction in the severity of clinical symptoms

In summary, probiotics have an anti-inflammatory effect on psoriasis and atopic dermatitis, decreasing the severity of the disease symptoms.

References

Abdelhadi S., Nordlind K., Johansson B. et al. Expression of calcitonin gene-related peptide in atopic dermatitis and correlation with distress. Immunopharmacol Immunotoxicol 2024; 46(1): 67–72.

Abrahamsson T.R., Jakobsson T., Böttcher M.F. et al. Probiotics in prevention of IgE-associated eczema: a double-blind, randomized, placebo-controlled trial. J Allergy Clin Immunol 2007; 119(5); 1174–1180.

Afifi L., Danesh M.J., Lee K.M. et al. Dietary behaviors in psoriasis: patient-reported outcomes from a U.S. National Survey. Dermatol Ther (Heidelb) 2017; 7(2): 227–242.

Aggarwal N., Kitano S., Puah G.R.Y. et al. Microbiome and human health: current understanding, engineering, and enabling technologies. Chem Rev 2023; 123(1): 31–72.

Agrawal R., Hu A., Bollag W.B. The skin and inflamm-aging. Biology 2023; 12(11): 1396.

Akbarzadeh A., Taheri M., Ebrahimi B. et al. Evaluation of Lactocare® synbiotic administration on the serum electrolytes and trace elements levels in psoriasis patients: a randomized, double-blind, placebo-controlled clinical trial study. Biol Trace Elem Res 2022; 200(10): 4230–4237.

Akerstrom U., Reitamo S., Langeland T. et al. Comparison of moisturizing creams for the prevention of atopic dermatitis relapse: a randomized double-blind controlled multicentre clinical trial. Acta Derm Venereol 2015; 95(5): 587–592.

Albèr C., Buraczewska-Norin I., Kocherbitov V. et al. Effects of water activity and low molecular weight humectants on skin permeability and hydration dynamics — a double-blind, randomized and controlled study. Int J Cosmet Sci 2014; 36(5): 412–418.

Al-Mutairi A., Elkashlan M. Nail psoriasis treated with pulse dye laser. Indian J Dermatol 2013; 58(3): 243.

Alora M.B., Anderson R.R., Quinn T.R., Taylor C.R. CO_2-laser resurfacing of psoriatic plaques: a pilot study. Lasers Surg Med 1998; 22(3): 165–170.

Alzahrani S.A., Alzamil F.M., Aljuhni A.M. et al. A systematic review evaluating the effectiveness of several biological therapies for the treatment of skin psoriasis. Cureus 2023; 15(12): e50588.

Amaro-Ortiz A., Yan B., D'Orazio J.A. Ultraviolet radiation, aging and the skin: prevention of damage by topical cAMP manipulation. Molecules 2014; 19(5): 6202–6219.

Angelova-Fischer I., Rippke F., Richter D. et al. Stand-alone emollient treatment reduces flares after discontinuation of topical steroid treatment in atopic dermatitis: a double-blind, randomized, vehicle-controlled, left-right comparison study. Acta Derm Venereol 2018; 98(5): 517–523.

Arndt J., Smith N., Tausk F. Stress and atopic dermatitis. Curr Allergy Asthma Rep 2008; 8(4): 312–317.

Arnone M., Takahashi M.D.F., Carvalho A.V.E. et al. Diagnostic and therapeutic guidelines for plaque psoriasis — Brazilian Society of Dermatology. An Bras Dermatol 2019; 94(2 Suppl 1): 76–107.

Arrieta M.C., Stiemsma L.T., Amenyogbe N. et al. The intestinal microbiome in early life: health and disease. Front Immunol 2014; 5: 427.

Ashida Y., Denda M. Dry environment increases mast cell number and histamine content in dermis in hairless mice. Br J Dermatol. 2003; 149(2): 240–247.

Bak H., Hong S.P., Jeong S.K. et al. Altered epidermal lipid layers induced by long-term exposure to suberythemal-dose ultraviolet. Int J Dermatol 2011; 50(7): 832–837.

Barcelos R.C., Vey L.T., Segat H.J. et al. Influence of trans fat on skin damage in first-generation rats exposed to UV radiation. Photochem Photobiol 2015; 91(2): 424–430.

Barrea L., Balato N., Di Somma C. et al. Nutrition and psoriasis: is there any association between the severity of the disease and adherence to the Mediterranean diet? J Transl Med 2015; 13: 18.

Barton M., Sidbury R. Advances in understanding and managing atopic dermatitis. F1000Res 2015; 4: F1000 Faculty Rev-1296.

Baurecht H., Ruhlemann M.C., Rodriguez E. et al. Epidermal lipid composition, barrier integrity, and eczematous inflammation are associated with skin microbiome configuration. J Allergy Clin Immunol 2018; 141(5): 1668–1676.

Benhadou F., Mintoff D., Del Marmol V. Psoriasis: keratinocytes or immune cells — which is the trigger? Dermatol 2019; 235(2): 91–100.

Best K.P., Gold M., Kennedy D. et al. Omega-3 long-chain PUFA intake during pregnancy and allergic disease outcomes in the offspring: a systematic review and meta-analysis of observational studies and randomized controlled trials. Am J Clin Nutr 2016; 103(1): 128–143.

Bhawan J., Oh C.H., Lew R. et al. Histopathologic differences in the photoaging process in facial versus arm skin. Am J Dermatopathol 1992; 14(3): 224–230.

Biniek K., Levi K., Dauskardt R.H. Solar UV radiation reduces the barrier function of human skin. Proc Natl Acad Sci USA 2012; 109(42): 17111–17116.

Blank I.H. Factors which influence the water content of the stratum corneum. J Invest Dermatol 1952; 18(6): 433–440.

Bleizgys A. Vitamin D dosing: basic principles and a brief algorithm (2021 Update). Nutrients 2021; 13(12): 4415.

Boelsma E., van de Vijver L.P., Goldbohm R.A. et al. Human skin condition and its associations with nutrient concentrations in serum and diet. Am J Clin Nutrition 2003; 77(2): 348–355.

Bolla B.S., Erdei L., Urbán E. Cutibacterium acnes regulates the epidermal barrier properties of HPV-KER human immortalized keratinocyte cultures. Sci Rep 2020; 10(1): 12815.

Bożek A., Reich A. The reliability of three psoriasis assessment tools: psoriasis area and severity index, body surface area and physician global assessment. Adv Clin Exp Med 2017; 26(5): 851–856.

Bruno M., Strober B., Del Rosso J.Q. Topical management of plaque psoriasis — a review and case series discussion with focus on aryl hydrocarbon receptor modulation. J Clin Aesthet Dermatol 2023; 16(9 Suppl 1): S3–S12.

Buhaş M.C., Gavrilaş L.I., Candrea R. et al. Gut microbiota in psoriasis. Nutrients 2022; 14(14): 2970.

Buhr E.D., Takahashi J.S. Molecular components of the Mammalian circadian clock. Handb Exp Pharmacol 2013; 217: 3–27.

Buske-Kirschbaum A., Ebrecht M., Kern S., Hellhammer D.H. Endocrine stress responses in TH1-mediated chronic inflammatory skin disease (psoriasis vulgaris) — do they parallel stress-induced endocrine changes in TH2-mediated inflammatory dermatoses (atopic dermatitis)? Psychoneuroendocrinology 2006; 31(4): 439–446.

Camargo C.A. Jr., Ganmaa D., Sidbury R. et al. Randomized trial of vitamin D supplementation for winter-related atopic dermatitis in children. J Allergy Clin Immuno 2014; 134(4): 831–835.

Camilion J.V., Khanna S., Anasseri S. et al. Physiological, pathological, and circadian factors impacting skin hydration. Cureus 2022; 14(8): e27666.

Carbajo J.M., Maraver F. Salt water and skin interactions: new lines of evidence. Int J Biometeorol 2018; 62(8): 1345–1360.

Căruntu C., Boda D., Musat S. et al. Stress-induced mast cell activation in glabrous and hairy skin. Mediators Inflamm 2014; 2014: 105950.

Celakovska J., Ettlerova K., Ettler K. et al. Evaluation of cow's milk allergy in a large group of adolescent and adult patients with atopic dermatitis. Acta Medica (Hradec Kralove) 2012; 55(3): 125–129.

Celakovska J., Ettlerova K., Ettler K. et al. The effect of wheat allergy on the course of atopic eczema in patients over 14 years of age. Acta Medica (Hradec Kralove) 2011a; 54(4): 157–162.

Celakovska J., Ettlerova K., Ettler K., Vaneckova J. Egg allergy in patients over 14 years old suffering from atopic eczema. Int J Dermatol 2011b; 50(7): 811–818.

Cepeda A.M., Del Giacco S.R., Villalba S. et al. A traditional diet is associated with a reduced risk of eczema and wheeze in Colombian children. Nutrients 2015; 7(7): 5098–5110.

Çetinarslan T., Kümper L., Fölster-Holst R. The immunological and structural epidermal barrier dysfunction and skin microbiome in atopic dermatitis — an update. Front Mol Biosc 2023; 10: 1159404.

Chang Y., Trivedi M.K., Jha A. et al. Synbiotics for prevention and treatment of atopic dermatitis: a meta-analysis of randomized clinical trials. JAMA Pediatr 2016; 170(3): 236–242.

Chapman S.J., Walsh A. Desmosomes, corneosomes and desquamation. An ultrastructural study of adult pig epidermis. Arch Dermatol Res 1990; 282(5): 304–310.

Chiang C., Eichenfield L.F. Quantitative assessment of combination bathing and moisturizing regimens on skin hydration in atopic dermatitis. Pediatr Dermatol 2009; 26(3): 273–278.

Choi H.K., Cho Y.H., Lee E.O. et al. Phytosphingosine enhances moisture level in human skin barrier through stimulation of the filaggrin biosynthesis and degradation leading to NMF formation. Arch Dermatol Res 2017; 309(10): 795–803.

Choi J.Y., Owusu-Ayim M., Dawe R. et al. Narrowband Ultraviolet B phototherapy is associated with a reduction in topical corticosteroid and clinical improvement in atopic dermatitis: a historical inception cohort study. Clin Exp Dermatol 2021; 46(6): 1067–1074.

Choi S.M., Lee B.M. Safety and risk assessment of ceramide 3 in cosmetic products. Food Chem Toxicol 2015; 84: 8–17.

Chovatiya R., Silverberg J.I. Pathophysiology of atopic dermatitis and psoriasis: implications for management in children. Children (Basel) 2019; 6(10): 108.

Chu H., Shin J.U., Lee J. et al. Successful treatment of lichen amyloidosis accompanied by atopic dermatitis by fractional CO_2 laser. J Cosmet Laser Ther 2017; 19(6): 345–346.

Çiçek F., Köle M.T. Evaluation of the impact of serum vitamin D levels on the scoring atopic dermatitis index in pediatric atopic dermatitis. Children (Basel) 2023; 10(9): 1522.

Clausen M.L., Edslev S.M., Andersen P.S. et al. Staphylococcus aureus colonization in atopic eczema and its association with filaggrin gene mutations. Br J Dermatol 2017; 177(5): 1394–1400.

Cundell A.M. Microbial ecology of the human skin. Microb Ecol 2018; 76(1): 113–120.

Czarnowicki T., Krueger J.G., Guttman-Yassky E. Novel concepts of prevention and treatment of atopic dermatitis through barrier and immune manipulations with implications for the atopic march. J Allergy Clin Immunol 2017; 139(6): 1723–1734.

Dai Q., Zhang Y., Liu Q., Zhang C. Efficacy and safety of vitamin D supplementation on psoriasis: a systematic review and meta-analysis. PLoS One 2023; 18(11): e0294239.

Danso M.O., Boiten W., van Drongelen V. et al. Altered expression of epidermal lipid bio-synthesis enzymes in atopic dermatitis skin is accompanied by changes in stratum corneum lipid composition. J. Dermatol Sci 2017; 88(1): 57–66.

Darlenski R., Hristakieva E., Aydin U. et al. Epidermal barrier and oxidative stress parameters improve during in 311 nm narrow band UVB phototherapy of plaque type psoriasis. J Dermatol Sci 2018; 91(1): 28–34.

Darmstadt G.L., Ahmed S., Ahmed A.S., Saha S.K. Mechanism for prevention of infection in preterm neonates by topical emollients: a randomized, controlled clinical trial. Pediatr Infect Dis J 2014; 33(11): 1124–1127.

David M., Efron D., Hodak E., Even-Paz Z. Treatment of psoriasis at the Dead Sea: Why, how and when? Isr Med Assoc J 2000; 2(3): 232–234.

De Arruda L.H., De Moraes A.P. The impact of psoriasis on quality of life. Br J Dermatol 2001; 144(58): 33–36.

De Leeuw J., Tank B., Bjerring P.J. Concomitant treatment of psoriasis of the hands and feet with pulsed dye laser and topical calcipotriol, salicylic acid, or both: a prospective open study in 41 patients. J Am Acad Dermatol 2006; 54(2): 266–271.

De Leeuw J., Van Lingen R.G., Both H. et al. A comparative study on the efficacy of treatment with 585-nm pulsed dye laser and ultraviolet B-TL01 in plaque type psoriasis. Dermatol Surg 2009; 35(1): 80–91.

de Macedo G.M., Nunes S., Barreto T. Skin disorders in diabetes mellitus: an epidemiology and physiopathology review. Diabetol Metab Syndr 2016; 8(1): 63.

de Miranda R.B., Weimer P., Rossi R.C. Effects of hydrolyzed collagen supplementation on skin aging: a systematic review and meta-analysis. Int J Dermatol 2021; 60(12): 1449–1461.

De Pessemier B., Grine L., Debaere M. et al. Gut-skin axis: current knowledge of the interrelationship between microbial dysbiosis and skin conditions. Microorganisms 2021; 9(2): 353.

Debbaneh M.G., Levin E., Sanchez Rodriguez R. et al. Plaque-based sub-blistering dosimetry: reaching PASI-75 after two treatments with 308-nm excimer laser in a generalized psoriasis patient. J Dermatol Treat 2015; 26(1): 45–48.

Denda M., Sato J., Tsuchiya T. et al. Low humidity stimulates epidermal DNA synthesis and amplifies the hyperproliferative response to barrier disruption: implication for seasonal exacerbations of inflammatory dermatoses. J Invest Dermatol 1998; 111(5): 873–878.

Dewi D.A.R., Arimuko A., Norawati L. et al. Exploring the impact of hydrolyzed collagen oral supplementation on skin rejuvenation: a systematic review and meta-analysis. Cureus 2023; 15(12): e50231.

Di Marzio L., Centi C., Cinque B. et al. Effect of the lactic acid bacterium Streptococcus thermophilus on stratum corneum ceramide levels and signs and symptoms of atopic dermatitis patients. Exp Dermatol 2003; 12(5): 615–620.

Di Marzio L., Cinque B., Cupelli F. et al. Increase of skin-ceramide levels in aged subjects following a short-term topical application of bacterial sphingomyelinase from Streptococcus thermophilus. Int J Immunopathol Pharmacol 2008; 21(1): 137–143.

Disphanurat W., Viarasilpa W., Chakkavittumrong P. et al. The clinical effect of oral vitamin D2 supplementation on psoriasis: a double-blind, randomized, placebo-controlled study. Dermatol Res Pract 2019; 2019: 5237642.

Dixon K.M., Tongkao-On W., Sequeira V.B. et al. Vitamin D and death by sunshine. Int J Mol Sci 2013; 14(1): 1964–1977.

Dolan K.E., Pizano J.M., Gossard C.M. et al. Probiotics and disease: a comprehensive summary — part 6, skin health. Integr Med (Encinitas) 2017; 16(4): 32–41.

Draelos Z.D. Nutrition and enhancing youthful-appearing skin. Clin Dermatol 2020; 38(5): 582–586.

Draelos Z.D. The science behind skin care: moisturizers. J Cosmet Dermatol 2018; 17(2): 138–144.

Drago L., Lemoli E., Rodighiero V. et al. Effects of Lactobacillus salivarius LS01 (DSM 22775) treatment on adult atopic dermatitis: a randomized placebo-controlled study. Int J Immunopathol Pharmacol 2011; 24(4): 1037–1048.

Drew G.S. Psoriasis. Prim Care 2009; 23(2): 385–406.

Dumas M., Sadick N.S., Noblesse E. et al. Hydrating skin by stimulating biosynthesis of aquaporins. J Drugs Dermatol 2007; 6(6 Suppl): S20–S24.

Eichenfield L.F., Tom W.L., Berger T.G. et al. Guidelines of care for the management of atopic dermatitis: Section 2. Management and treatment of atopic dermatitis with topical therapies. J Am Acad Dermatol 2014; 71(1): 116–132.

Elenkov I.J., Chrousos G.P. Stress hormones, Th1/Th2 patterns, pro/antiinflamma-tory cytokines and susceptibility to disease. Trends Endocrinol Metab 1999; 10(9): 359–368.

Elias M.S., Long H.A., Newman C.F. et al. Proteomic analysis of filaggrin deficiency identifies molecular signatures characteristic of atopic eczema. J Allergy Clin Immunol 2017; 140(5): 1299–1309.

Elias P.M. Optimizing emollient therapy for skin barrier repair in atopic dermatitis. Ann Allergy Asthma Immunol 2022; 128(5): 505–511.

Elias P.M. Stratum corneum defensive functions: an integrated view. J Invest Dermatol 2005; 125(2): 183–200.

Emer J. Platelet-rich plasma (PRP): current applications in dermatology. Skin Therapy Lett 2019; 24(5): 1–6.

Engebretsen K.A., Kezic S., Riethmüller C. et al. Changes in filaggrin degrada-tion products and corneocyte surface texture by season. Br J Dermatol 2018; 178(5): 1143–1150.

Eppinga H., Konstantinov S.R., Peppelenbosch M.P., Thio H.B. The microbiome and psoriatic arthritis. Curr Rheumatol Rep 2014; 16(3): 1–8.

Faber C., Ziboh V.A., Chapkin R.S. Role of omega-3 fatty acids in anti-inflammatory skin responses. J Lipid Res 2020; 61(5): 861–870.

Feingold K.R., Elias P.M. Role of lipids in the formation and maintenance of the cutaneous permeability barrier. Biochim Biophys Acta 2014; 1841(3): 280–294.

Feldman S.R., Mellen B.G., Housman T.S. et al. Efficacy of the 308-nm excimer laser for treatment of psoriasis: results of a multicenter study. J Am Acad Dermatol 2002; 46(6): 900–906.

Fernández-Guarino M., Harto A., Sánchez-Ronco M. et al. Pulsed dye laser vs. pho-todynamic therapy in the treatment of refractory nail psoriasis: a comparative pilot study. J Eur Acad Dermatol Venereol 2009; 23(8): 891–895.

Finamor D.C., Sinigaglia-Coimbra R., Neves L.C. et al. A pilot study assessing the effect of prolonged administration of high daily doses of vitamin D on the clinical course of vitiligo and psoriasis. Dermatoendocrinol 2013; 5(1): 222–234.

Firooz A., Zartab H., Sadr B. et al. Daytime changes of skin biophysical character-istics: a study of hydration, transepidermal water loss, pH, sebum, elasticity, erythema, and color index on Middle Eastern skin. Indian J Dermatol 2016; 61(6): 700.

Fleury O.M., McAleer M.A., Feuillie C. et al. Clumping factor B promotes adherence of Staphylococcus aureus to corneocytes in atopic dermatitis. Infect Immun 2017; 85(6): e00994-16.

Flores-Balderas X., Peña-Peña M., Rada K.M. et al. Beneficial effects of plant-based diets on skin health and inflammatory skin diseases. Nutrients 2023; 15(13): 2842.

Fowler J. Understanding the role of Natural Moisturizing Factor in skin hydration. Practical Dermatol 2012; July: 36–40.

Friedman A.J., von Grote E.C., Meckfessel M.H. Urea: a clinically oriented overview from bench to bedside. J Drugs Dermatol 2016; 15(5): 633–639.

Fujimura K.E., Slusher N.A., Cabana M.D., Lynch S.V. Role of the gut microbiota in defining human health. Exp Rev Anti-Infect Ther 2010; 8(4): 435–454.

Furuhashi T., Torii K., Kato H. et al. Efficacy of excimer light therapy (308 nm) for palmoplantar pustulosis with the induction of circulating regulatory T-cells. Exp Dermatol 2011; 20(9): 768–770.

Gallegos-Alcalá P., Jiménez M., Cervantes-García D., Salinas E. The keratinocyte as a crucial cell in the predisposition, onset, progression, therapy and study of the atopic dermatitis. Int J Mol Sci 2021; 22(19): 10661.

Gao T., Wang X., Li Y., Ren F. The role of probiotics in skin health and related gut–skin axis: a review. Nutrients 2023; 15(14): 3123.

Gattu S., Pang M.L., Pugashetti R. et al. Pilot evaluation of supra-erythemogenic phototherapy with excimer laser in the treatment of patients with moderate to severe plaque psoriasis. J Dermatolog Treat 2010; 21(1): 54–60.

Gazerani P. Antipruritic effects of botulinum neurotoxins. Toxins (Basel) 2018; 10(4): 143.

Gerdes S., Campanati A., Ratzinger G. et al. Improvements in plaque psoriasis associated with calcipotriol/betamethasone aerosol foam treatment: a post hoc analysis of non-interventional studies and clinical experience. Dermatol Ther (Heidelb) 2024; 14(3): 793–804.

Gharib K., Mostafa A., Elsayed A. Evaluation of botulinum toxin type A injection in the treatment of localized chronic pruritus. J Clin Aesthet Dermatol 2020; 13(12): 12–17.

Giménez-Arnau A. Standards for the protection of skin barrier function. Curr Probl Dermatol 2016; 49: 123–134.

Gisondi P., Rossini M., Di Cesare A. et al. Vitamin D status in patients with chronic plaque psoriasis. Br J Dermatol 2012; 166(3): 505–510.

Glatz M., Jo J.H., Kennedy E.A. et al. Emollient use alters skin barrier and microbes in infants at risk for developing atopic dermatitis. PLoS One 2018; 13(2): e0192443.

Göblös A., Varga E., Farkas K. et al. Genetic Investigation of Inverse Psoriasis. Life (Basel). 2021; 11(7): 654.

Goldberg D.J. (Ed.) Procedures in Cosmetic Dermatology Series: Lasers and Lights: Volume 1: Text with DVD: Vascular, Pigmentation, Scars, Medical Applications. Saunders, 2005.

Göllner I., Voss W., von Hehn U., Kammerer S. Ingestion of an oral hyaluronan solution improves skin hydration, wrinkle reduction, elasticity, and skin roughness: results of a clinical study. J Evid Based Complementary Altern Med 2017; 2294: 816–823.

Gonzalez M.E., Schaffer J.V., Orlow S.J. et al. Cutaneous microbiome effects of fluticasone propionate cream and adjunctive bleach baths in childhood atopic dermatitis. J Am Acad Dermatol 2016; 75(3): 481–493.

Grän F., Kerstan A., Serfling E. et al. Current developments in the immunology of psoriasis. Yale J Biol Med 2020; 93(1): 97–110.

Green H. The role of calcium in epidermal barrier function. J Dermatol Sci 1999; 10(1): 3–7.

Grether-Beck S., Felsner I., Brenden H. et al. Urea uptake enhances barrier function and antimicrobial defense in humans by regulating epidermal gene expression. J Invest Dermatol 2012; 132(6): 1561–1572.

Grice E.A., Kong H.H., Conlan S. et al. Topographical and temporal diversity of the human skin microbiome. Science 2009; 324: 1190–1192.

Groeger D., O'Mahony L., Murphy E.F. et al. Bifidobacterium infantis 35624 modulates host inflammatory processes beyond the gut. Gut Microbes 2013; 4(4): 325–339.

Guibas G.V., Makris M., Chliva C. et al. Atopic dermatitis, food allergy and dietary interventions. A tale of controversy. An Bras Dermatol 2013; 88(5): 839–841.

Gutman A.B., Kligman A.M., Sciacca J. et al. Soak and smear. A standard technique revisited. Arch Dermatol 2005; 141(12): 1556–1559.

Hajar T., Hanifin J.M., Tofte S.J., Simpson E.L. Prehydration is effective for rapid control of recalcitrant atopic dermatitis. Dermatitis 2014; 25(2): 56–59.

Halevy S., Giryes H., Friger M., Sukenik S. Dead Sea bath salt for the treatment of psoriasis vulgaris: a double-blind controlled study. Eur J Acad Dermatol Venereol 1997; 9: 237–242.

Hanifin J.M., Rajka G. Diagnostic features of atopic dermatitis. Acta Derm Venereol (Stockh) 1980; 92(Suppl): 44–47.

Harari M., Shani J. Demographic evaluation of successful antipsoriatic climatotherapy at the Dead Sea (Israel) DMZ Clinic. Int J Dermatol 1997; 36(4): 304–308.

Harris-Tryon T.A., Grice E.A. Microbiota and maintenance of skin barrier function. Science 2022; 376(6569): 940–945.

Hashim P.W., Nia J.K., Terrano D. et al. A comparative study to evaluate epidermal barrier integrity of psoriasis patients treated with calcipotriene/betamethasone topical suspension versus betamethasone dipropionate 0.05% lotion. J Drugs Dermatol 2017; 16(8): 747–752.

Hattangdi-Haridas S.R., Lanham-New S.A., Wong W.H.S. et al. Vitamin D deficiency and effects of vitamin D supplementation on disease severity in patients with atopic dermatitis: a systematic review and meta-analysis in adults and children. Nutrients 2019; 11(8): 1854.

Heckmann M., Teichmann B., Pause B.M., Plewig G. Botulinum toxin type A injection in the treatment of lichen simplex: a pilot study. J Am Acad Dermatol 2002; 46(4): 617–619.

Herrero-Fernandez M., Montero-Vilchez T., Diaz-Calvillo P. et al. Impact of water exposure and temperature changes on skin barrier function. J Clin Med 2022; 11(2): 298.

Hodak E., Gottlieb A.B., Segal T. et al. Climatotherapy at the Dead Sea is a remittive therapy for psoriasis: combined effects on epidermal and immunologic activation. J Am Acad Dermatol 2003; 49(3): 451–457.

Holick M.F., Binkley N.C., Bischoff-Ferrari H.A. et al. Evaluation, treatment, and prevention of vitamin D deficiency: an Endocrine Society clinical practice guideline. J Clin Endocrinol Metab 2011; 96(7): 1911–1930.

Hon K.L., Tsang Y.C., Lee V.W. et al. Efficacy of sodium hypochlorite (bleach) baths to reduce Staphylococcus aureus colonization in childhood-onset moderate-to-severe eczema: a randomized, placebo-controlled cross-over trial. J Dermatol Treat 2016; 27(2): 156–162.

Hong J., Malick F., Sivanesan P., Koo Y. Expanding use of the 308-nm excimer laser for the treatment of psoriasis. Practical Dermatol 2007; Apr: S13–S16.

Hrestak D., Matijašić M., Čipčić Paljetak H. et al. Skin microbiota in atopic dermatitis. Int J Mol Sci 2022; 23(7): 3503.

Hruza G.J. Excimer laser vs pulsed dye laser for psoriasis. J Watch 2005; 4(12): 521128.

Huang T.H., Lin C.F., Alalaiwe A. et al. Apoptotic or antiproliferative activity of natural products against keratinocytes for the treatment of psoriasis. Int J Mol Sci 2019; 20(10): 2558.

Inoue Y., Kambara T., Murata N. et al. Effects of oral administration of Lactobacillus acidophilus L-92 on the symptoms and serum cytokines of atopic dermatitis in Japanese adults: a double-blind, randomized, clinical trial. Int Arch Allergy Immunol 2015; 165(4); 247–254.

Inoue Y., Nakagawara R., Kambara T. et al. Prevalence of atopic dermatitis in Japanese infants treated with moisturizer since birth and its relation to FLG mutations. Eur J Dermatol 2013; 23(2): 288–289.

Inuzuka Y., Natsume O., Matsunaga M. et al. Washing with water alone versus soap in maintaining remission of eczema. Pediatr Int 2020; 62(6): 663–668.

Jacobi A., Mayer A., Augustin M. Keratolytics and emollients and their role in the therapy of psoriasis: a systematic review. Dermatol Ther (Heidelb) 2015; 5(1): 1–18.

James-Smith M.A., Hellner B., Annunziato N., Mitragotri S. Effect of surfactant mixtures on skin structure and barrier properties. Ann Biomed Eng 2011; 39(4): 1215–1223.

Jensen K.K., Serup J., Alsing K.K. Psoriasis and seasonal variation: a systematic review on reports from Northern and Central Europe — Little overall variation but distinctive subsets with improvement in summer or wintertime. Skin Res Technol 2022; 28(1): 180–186.

Jeong K., Kim M., Jeon S.A. et al. A randomized trial of Lactobacillus rhamnosus IDCC 3201 tyndallizate (RHT3201) for treating atopic dermatitis. Pediatr Allergy Immunol 2020; 31(7): 783–792.

Jeskey J., Kurien C., Blunk H. et al. Atopic dermatitis: a review of diagnosis and treatment. J Pediatr Pharmacol Ther 2024; 29(6): 587–603.

Jiminez V., Yusuf N. Bacterial metabolites and inflammatory skin diseases. Metabolites 2023; 13(8): 952.

Johnson A.M.F., DePaolo R.W. Window-of-opportunity: neonatal gut microbiota and atopy. Hepatobiliary Surg Nutr 2017; 6(3): 190–192.

Kaczmarski M., Cudowska B., Sawicka-Żukowska M., Bobrus-Chociej A. Supplementation with long chain polyunsaturated fatty acids in treatment of atopic dermatitis in children. Postep Derm Alergol 2013; 30(2): 103–107.

Kaikiri H., Miyamoto J., Kawakami T. et al. Supplemental feeding of a gut microbial metabolite of linoleic acid, 10-hydroxy-cis-12-octadecenoic acid, alleviates spontaneous atopic dermatitis and modulates intestinal microbiota in NC/Nga mice. Int J Food Sci Nutr 2017; 68(8): 941–951.

Kalashnikova N.G. Treatment of skin manifestations of psoriasis by spatially modulated ablation. Vestnik Esteticheskoi Meditsini 2014; 13(3–4): 105–112.

Kamangar F., Koo J., Heller M. et al. Oral vitamin D, still a viable treatment option for psoriasis. J Dermatol Treat 2013; 24(4): 261–267.

Katagiri C., Sato J., Nomura J., Denda M. Changes in environmental humidity affect the water-holding property of the stratum corneum and its free amino acid content, and the expression of filaggrin in the epidermis of hairless mice. J Dermatol Sci. 2003; 31(1): 29–35.

Katoh N., Ohya Y., Ikeda M. et al. Japanese guidelines for atopic dermatitis 2020. Allergol Int 2020; 69(3): 356–369.

Katz U., Shoenfeld Y., Zakin V. et al. Scientific evidence of the therapeutic effects of Dead Sea treatments: a systematic review. Semin Arthritis Rheum 2012; 42(2): 186–200.

Khattab F.M. Evaluation of botulinum toxin A as an optional treatment for atopic dermatitis. J Clin Aesthet Dermatol 2020; 13(7): 32–35.

Kierasińska M., Donskow-Łysoniewska K. Both the microbiome and the macrobiome can influence immune responsiveness in psoriasis. Central Eur J Immunol 2021; 46(4): 502–508.

Kim H.J., Kim H.Y., Lee S.Y. et al. Clinical efficacy and mechanism of probiotics in allergic diseases. Korean J Pediatr 2013; 56(9): 369–376.

Kim H.S., Yosipovitch G. The skin microbiota and itch: is there a link? J Clin Med 2020; 9(4): 1190.

Kim J., Kim M., Shin H. The omega-3/omega-6 ratio and its impact on the skin's barrier function and hydration. J Derm Sci 2018; 92(4): 287–293.

Kim J.E., Kim H.J., Lew B.L. et al. Consensus guidelines for the treatment of atopic dermatitis in Korea (Part I): general management and topical treatment. Ann Dermatol 2015; 27(5): 563–577.

Kim J.E., Kim H.S. Microbiome of the skin and gut in atopic dermatitis (AD): understanding the pathophysiology and finding novel management strategies. J Clin Med 2019; 8(4): 444.

Kim J.H., Son S.M., Park H. et al. Taxonomic profiling of skin microbiome and correlation with clinical skin parameters in healthy Koreans. Sci Rep 2021; 11(1): 16269.

Kim S., Park J.W., Yeon Y. et al. Influence of exposure to summer environments on skin properties. J Eur Acad Dermatol Venereol 2019; 33(1): 2192–2196.

Kim W.K., Han D.H., Jang Y.J. et al. Alleviation of DSS-induced colitis via Lactobacillus acidophilus treatment in mice. Food Funct 2021; 12(1): 340–350.

Kim Y., Lim K.M. Skin barrier dysfunction and filaggrin. Arch Pharm Res 2021; 44(1): 36–48.

Kircik L.H. Why do we need another moisturizer for our acne patients? J Drugs Dermatol 2014; 13(8): S88.

Klaassens E.S., Boesten R.J., Haarman M. et al. Mixed-species genomic microarray analysis of fecal samples reveals differential transcriptional responses of bifidobacteria in breast- and formula-fed infants. App Environ Microbiol 2009; 75(9): 2668–2676.

Koh L.F., Ong R.Y., Common J.E. Skin microbiome of atopic dermatitis. Allergol Int 2022; 71(1): 31–39.

Kong H.H., Oh J., Deming C. et al. Temporal shifts in the skin microbiome associated with disease flares and treatment in children with atopic dermatitis. Genome Res 2012; 22(5): 850–859.

Kouda K., Tanaka T., Kouda M. et al. Low-energy diet in atopic dermatitis patients: clinical findings and DNA damage. J Physiol Anthropol Appl Human Sci 2000; 19(5): 225–228.

Krueger G., Koo J., Lebwohl M. et al. The impact of psoriasis on quality of life: results of a 1998 National Psoriasis Foundation patient-membership survey. Arch Dermatol 2001; 137(3): 280–284.

Kubanov A.A., Karamova A.E., Znamenskaya I.F. et al. PASI (Psoriasis Area and Severity Index) in the evaluation of the clinical manifestations of psoriasis. Vestnik Dermatologii i Venerologii 2016; 4: 33–38.

Kukkonen K., Savilahti E., Haahtela T. et al. Probiotics and prebiotic galacto-oligosaccharides in the prevention of allergic diseases: a randomized, double-blind, placebo-controlled trial. J Allergy Clin Immunol 2007; 119(1): 192–198.

Kwon M.S., Lim S.K., Jang J.Y. et al. Lactobacillus sakei WIKIM30 ameliorates atopic dermatitis-like skin lesions by inducing regulatory T cells and altering gut microbiota structure in mice. Front Immunol 2018; 9: 1905.

Kwon T.R., Oh C.T., Choi E.J. et al. Conditioned medium from human bone marrow-derived mesenchymal stem cells promotes skin moisturization and effacement of wrinkles in UVB-irradiated SKH-1 hairless mice. Photodermatol Photoimmunol Photomed 2016; 32(3): 120–128.

Langan S.M., Irvine A.D., Weidinger S. Atopic dermatitis. Lancet 2020; 396(10247): 345–360.

Lebeer S., Vanderleyden J., De Keersmaecker S.C. Host interactions of probiotic bacterial surface molecules: comparison with commensals and pathogens. Nat Rev Microbiol 2010; 8(3): 171–184.

Lebwohl M. The role of salicylic acid in the treatment of psoriasis. Int J Dermatol 1999; 38(1): 16–24.

Lebwohl M., Menter A., Weiss J. et al. Calcitriol 3 microg/g ointment in the management of mild to moderate plaque type psoriasis: results from 2 placebo-controlled, multicenter, randomized double-blind, clinical studies. J Drugs Dermatol 2007; 6(4): 428–435.

Lee D.E., Huh C.S., Ra J. et al. Clinical evidence of effects of Lactobacillus plantarum HY7714 on skin aging: a randomized, double blind, placebo-controlled study. J Microbiol Biotechnol 2015; 25(12): 2160–2168.

Lee S.E., Lee S.H. Skin barrier and calcium. Ann Dermatol 2018; 30(3): 265–275.

Lee S.Y., Lee E., Park Y.M., Hong S.J. Microbiome in the gut–skin axis in atopic dermatitis. Allergy Asthma Immunol Res 2018; 10(4): 354–362.

Lee Y., Je Y.J., Lee S.S. et al. Changes in transepidermal water loss and skin hydration according to expression of aquaporin-3 in psoriasis. Ann Dermatol 2012; 24(2): 168–174.

Levin J., Friedlander S.F., Del Rosso J.Q. Atopic dermatitis and the stratum corneum. Part 2: other structural and functional characteristics of the stratum corneum barrier in atopic skin. J Clin Aesthet Dermatol 2013; 6(11): 49–54.

Lew L.C., Liong M.T. Bioactives from probiotics for dermal health: functions and benefits. J Appl Microbiol 2013; 114(5): 1241–1253.

Li S., Villarreal M., Stewart S. et al. Altered composition of epidermal lipids correlates with Staphylococcus aureus colonization status in atopic dermatitis. Br J Dermatol 2017; 177(4): e125–e127.

Liang X., Ou C., Zhuang J. et al. Interplay between skin microbiota dysbiosis and the host immune system in psoriasis: potential pathogenesis. Front Immunol 2021; 12: 764384.

Libon F., Courtois J., Le Goff C. et al. Sunscreens block cutaneous vitamin D production with only a minimal effect on circulating 25-hydroxyvitamin D. Arch Osteoporos 2017; 12(1): 66.

Lin C., Zeng T., Deng Y. et al. Treatment of psoriasis vulgaris using Bacteroides fragilis BF839: a single-arm, open preliminary clinical study. Sheng Wu Gong Cheng Xue Bao 2021; 37(11): 3828–3835.

Lone A.G., Atci E., Renslow R. et al. Staphylococcus aureus induces hypoxia and cellular damage in porcine dermal explants. Infect Immun 2015; 83(6): 2531–2541.

Lourencetti M., Abreu M.M. Use of active metabolites of vitamin D orally for the treatment of psoriasis. Rev Assoc Med Bras 2018; 64(7): 643–648. `

Luger T., Seite S., Humbert P. et al. Recommendations for adjunctive basic skin care in patients with psoriasis. Eur J Dermatol 2014; 24(2): 194–200.

Lyons A.B., Moy L., Moy R., Tung R. Circadian rhythm and the skin: a review of the literature. J Clin Aesthet Dermatol 2019; 12(9): 42–45.

Maarouf M., Hendricks A.J., Shi V.Y. Bathing additives for atopic dermatitis — a systematic review. Dermatitis 2019; 30(3): 191–197.

Marcheva B., Ramsey K.M., Peek C.B. et al. Circadian clocks and metabolism. Handb Exp Pharmacol 2013; 217: 127–155.

Matsumoto M., Ebata T., Hirooka J. et al. Antipruritic effects of the probiotic strain LKM512 in adults with atopic dermatitis. Ann Allergy Asthma Immunol 2014; 113(2): 209–216.

Matsunaga N., Itcho K., Hamamura K. et al. 24-hour rhythm of aquaporin-3 function in the epidermis is regulated by molecular clocks. J Invest Dermatol 2014; 134(6): 1636–1644.

Mattozzi C., Paolino G., Richetta A.G., Calvieri S. Psoriasis, vitamin D and the importance of the cutaneous barrier's integrity: an update. J Dermatol 2016; 43(5): 507–514.

Miajlovic H., Fallon P.G., Irvine A.D., Foster T.J. Effect of filaggrin breakdown products on growth of and protein expression by Staphylococcus aureus. J Allergy Clin Immunol 2010; 126(6): 1184–1190.

Miyake Y., Sasaki S., Tanaka K. et al. Dairy food, calcium and vitamin D intake in pregnancy, and wheeze and eczema in infants. Eur Respir J 2010; 35(6): 1228–1234.

Mizawa M., Yamaguchi M., Ueda C. et al. Stress evaluation in adult patients with atopic dermatitis using salivary cortisol. BioMed Res Int 2013; 2013: 138027.

Mojumdar E.H., Sparr E. The effect of pH and salt on the molecular structure and dynamics of the skin. Colloids Surf B Biointerfaces 2021; 198: 111476.

Moludi J., Khedmatgozar H., Saiedi S. et al. Probiotic supplementation improves clinical outcomes and quality of life indicators in patients with plaque psoriasis: a randomized double-blind clinical trial. Clin Nutr ESPEN 2021; 46: 33–39.

Moniaga C.S., Tominaga M., Takamori K. An altered skin and gut microbiota are involved in the modulation of itch in atopic dermatitis. Cells 2022; 11(23): 3930.

Moosazadeh M., Damiani G., Khademloo M. et al. Comparing vitamin D level between patients with psoriasis and healthy individuals: a systematic review and meta-analysis. J Evid Based Integr Med 2023; 28: 2515690X231211663.

Mori N., Kano M., Masuoka N. et al. Effect of probiotic and prebiotic fermented milk on skin and intestinal conditions in healthy young female students. Biosci Microbiota Food Health 2016; 35(3): 105–112.

Morison W.L., Atkinson D.F., Werthman L. Effective treatment of scalp psoriasis using the excimer (308 nm) laser. Photodermatol Photoimmunol Photomed 2006; 22(4): 181–183.

Moynihan J.A. Mechanisms of stress-induced modulation of immunity. Brain Behav Immun 2003; 17(Suppl 1): S11–S16.

Mudigonda T., Dabade T.S., Feldman S.R. A review of targeted ultraviolet B phototherapy for psoriasis. J Am Acad Dermatol 2012a; 66(4): 664–672.

Mudigonda T., Dabade T.S., West C.E., Feldman S.R. Therapeutic modalities for localized psoriasis: 308-nm UVB excimer laser versus nontargeted phototherapy. Cutis 2012b; 90(3): 149–154.

Mutanu Jungersted J., Hellgren L.I., Høgh J.K. et al. Ceramides and barrier function in healthy skin. Acta Derm Venereol 2010; 90(4): 350–353.

Myles I.A., Castillo C.R., Barbian K.D. et al. Therapeutic responses to Roseomonas mucosa in atopic dermatitis may involve lipid-mediated TNF-related epithelial repair. Sci Transl Med 2020; 12(560): eaaz8631.

Nagpal S., Na S., Na S., Rathnachalam R. Noncalcemic actions of vitamin D receptor ligands. Endocr Rev 2005; 26(5): 662–687.

Nakahigashi K., Kabashima K., Ikoma A. et al. Upregulation of aquaporin-3 is involved in keratinocyte proliferation and epidermal hyperplasia. J Invest Dermatol 2011; 131(4): 865–873.

Namazi M.R. Nicotinamide: a potential addition to the anti-psoriatic weaponry. FASEB J 2003; 17(11): 1377–1379.

Nasrollahi S.A., Ayatollahi A., Yazdanparast T. et al. Comparison of linoleic acid-containing water-in-oil emulsion with urea-containing water-in-oil emulsion in the treatment of atopic dermatitis: a randomized clinical trial. Clin Cosmet Investig Dermatol 2018; 11: 21–28.

Navarro-López V., Martínez-Andrés A., Ramírez-Boscá A. et al. Efficacy and safety of oral administration of a mixture of probiotic strains in patients with psoriasis: a randomized controlled clinical trial. Acta Derm Venereol 2019; 99(12): 1078–1084.

NICE Clinical Guidelines, No. 153, 2017. Psoriasis: assessment and management. https://www.nice.org.uk/guidance/cg153

Nomoto T., Iizaka S. Effect of an oral nutrition supplement containing collagen peptides on stratum corneum hydration and skin elasticity in hospitalized older adults: a multicenter open-label randomized controlled study. Adv Skin Wound Care 2020; 33(4): 186–191.

Noviello M.R., Italian Pediatric Group. Effects after daily use of washing products on infants aged 0–52 weeks. Minerva Pediatr 2005; 57(6): 411–418.

Nowicka D., Grywalska E. The role of immune defects and colonization of Staphylococcus aureus in the pathogenesis of atopic dermatitis. Anal Cell Pathol (Amst) 2018; 2018: 1956403.

Nylund L., Nermes M., Isolauri E. et al. Severity of atopic disease inversely correlates with intestinal microbiota diversity and butyrate-producing bacteria. Allergy 2015; 70(2): 241–244.

Oh J., Byrd A.L., Park M. et al. Temporal stability of the human skin microbiome. Cell 2016; 165(4): 854–866.

Okamoto N., Umehara K., Sonoda J. et al. Efficacy of the combined use of a mild foaming cleanser and moisturizer for the care of infant skin. Clin Cosmet Investig Dermatol 2017; 10: 393–401.

Olejniczak-Staruch I., Ciążyńska M., Sobolewska-Sztychny D. et al. Alterations of the skin and gut microbiome in psoriasis and psoriatic arthritis. Int J Mol Sci 2021; 22(8): 3998.

Ombra M.N., Paliogiannis P., Doneddu V. et al. Vitamin D status and risk for malignant cutaneous melanoma: recent advances. Eur J Cancer Prev 2017; 26(6): 532–541.

Oram Y., Karincaoğlu Y., Koyuncu E., Kaharaman F. Pulsed dye laser in the treatment of nail psoriasis. Dermatol Surg 2010; 36(3): 377–381.

Ortonne J., Chimenti S., Luger T. et al. Scalp psoriasis: European consensus on grading and treatment algorithm. J Eur Acad Dermatol Venereol 2009; 23(12): 1435–1444.

O'Toole A., Gooderham M. Topical roflumilast for plaque psoriasis. Skin Therapy Lett 2023; 28(5): 1–4.

Pagliaro M., Pecoraro L., Stefani C. et al. Bathing in atopic dermatitis in pediatric age: why, how and when. Pediatr Rep 2024; 16(1): 57–68.

Paller A.S., Kong H.H., Seed P. et al. The microbiome in patients with atopic dermatitis. J Allergy Clin Immunol 2019; 143(1): 26–35.

Pan M., Heinecke G., Bernardo S. et al. Urea: a comprehensive review of the clinical literature. Dermatol Online J 2013; 19(11): 20392.

Papakonstantinou E., Roth M., Karakiulakis G. Hyaluronic acid: a key molecule in skin aging. Dermatoendocrinol 2012; 4(3): 253–258.

Papp K.A., Thoning H., Gerdes S. et al. Matching-adjusted indirect comparison of efficacy outcomes in trials of calcipotriol plus betamethasone dipropionate foam and cream formulations for the treatment of plaque psoriasis. J Dermatolog Treat 2022; 33(7): 3005–3013.

Park K.K., Swan J., Koo J. Effective treatment of etanercept and phototherapy-resistant psoriasis using the excimer laser. Dermatol Online J 2012; 18(3): 2.

Park K.Y., Oh I.Y., Moon N.J., Seo S.J. Treatment of infraorbital dark circles in atopic dermatitis with a 2790-nm erbium: yttrium scandium gallium garnet laser: a pilot study. J Cosmet Laser Ther 2013; 15(2): 102–106.

Park S., Choi H.S., Bae J.H. Instant noodles, processed food intake, and dietary pattern are associated with atopic dermatitis in an adult population (KNHANES 2009–2011). Asia Pac J Clin Nutr 2016; 25(3): 602–613.

Park S.B., Im M., Lee Y. et al. Effect of emollients containing vegetable-derived Lactobacillus in the treatment of atopic dermatitis symptoms: split-body clinical trial. Ann Dermatol 2014; 26(2): 150–155.

Parrish J.A., Jaenicke K.F. Action spectrum for phototherapy of psoriasis. J Invest Dermatol 1981; 76(5): 359–362.

Patrick G.J., Archer N.K., Miller L.S. Which way do we go? Complex interactions in atopic dermatitis pathogenesis. J Invest Dermatol 2021; 141(2): 274–284.

Penders J., Thijs C., Vink C. et al. Factors influencing the composition of the intestinal microbiota in early infancy. Pediatrics 2006; 118(2): 511–521.

Perez A., Raab R., Chen T.C. et al. Safety and efficacy of oral calcitriol (1,25-dihydroxyvitamin D) for the treatment of psoriasis. Br J Dermatol 1996; 134(6): 1070–1078.

Phan C., Touvier M., Kesse-Guyot E. et al. Association between Mediterranean anti-inflammatory dietary profile and severity of psoriasis: results from the Nutri-Net-Santé cohort. JAMA Dermatol 2018; 154(9): 1017–1024.

Phiske M.M. Scalp psoriasis: a brief overview. J Cosmo Trichol 2016; 2: 110.

Proksch E., Berardesca E., Misery L. et al. Dry skin management: practical approach in light of latest research on skin structure and function. J Dermatolog Treat 2020; 31(7): 716–722.

Proksch E., Nissen H.P., Bremgartner M., Urquhart C. Bathing in a magnesium-rich Dead Sea salt solution improves skin barrier function, enhances skin hydration, and reduces inflammation in atopic dry skin. Int J Dermatol 2005; 44(2): 151–157.

Proksch E., Schunck M., Zague V. et al. Oral intake of specific bioactive collagen peptides reduces skin wrinkles and increases dermal matrix synthesis. Skin Pharmacol Physiol 2021; 34(6): 287–294.

Puebla-Barragan S., Reid G. Probiotics in cosmetic and personal care products: trends and challenges. Molecules 2021; 26(5): 1249.

Pullar J.M., Carr A.C., Vissers M.C.M. The roles of vitamin C in skin health. Nutrients 2017; 9(8): 866.

Queille-Roussel C., Hoffmann V., Ganslandt C. et al. Comparison of the antipsoriatic effect and tolerability of calcipotriol-containing products in the treatment of psoriasis vulgaris using a modified psoriasis plaque test. Clin Drug Investig 2012; 32(9): 613–619.

Radek K.A. Antimicrobial anxiety: the impact of stress on antimicrobial immunity. J Leukoc Biol 2010; 88(2): 263–277.

Rakita U., Kaundinya T., Silverberg J.I. Associations between shower and moisturizing practices with atopic dermatitis severity: a prospective longitudinal cohort study. Dermatitis 2023; 34(5): 425–431.

Ramírez-Boscá A., Navarro-López V., Martínez-Andrés A. et al. Identification of bacterial DNA in the peripheral blood of patients with active psoriasis. JAMA Dermatol 2015; 151(6): 670–671.

Rawlings A.V., Harding C.R. Moisturization and skin barrier function. Dermatol Ther 2004; 17(suppl 1): 43–48.

Rawlings A.V., Voegeli R. Stratum corneum proteases and dry skin conditions. Cell Tissue Res 2013; 351(2): 217–235.

Renert-Yuval Y., Del Duca E., Pavel A.B. et al. The molecular features of normal and atopic dermatitis skin in infants, children, adolescents, and adults. J Allergy Clin Immunol 2021; 148(1): 148–163.

Rinnerthaler M., Bischof J., Streubel M.K. et al. Oxidative stress in aging human skin. Biomolecules 2015; 5(2): 545–589.

Rogers J., Harding C., Mayo A. et al. Stratum corneum lipids: the effect of ageing and the seasons. Arch Dermatol Res 1996; 288(12): 765–770.

Russo E., Di Gloria L., Cerboneschi M. et al. Facial skin microbiome: aging-related changes and exploratory functional associations with host genetic factors, a pilot study. Biomedicines 2023; 11(3): 684.

Sakai S., Kikuchi K., Satoh J. et al. Functional properties of the stratum corneum in patients with diabetes mellitus: similarities to senile xerosis. Br J Dermatol 2005; 153(2): 319–323.

Salem I., Ramser A., Isham N., Ghannoum M.A. The gut microbiome as a major regulator of the gut–skin axis. Front Microbiol 2018; 9: 1459.

Schafer T., Bohler E., Ruhdorfer S. et al. Epidemiology of food allergy/food intolerance in adults: associations with other manifestations of atopy. Allergy 2001; 56(12): 1172–1179.

Schagen S.K., Zampeli V.A., Makrantonaki E., Zouboulis C.C. Discovering the link between nutrition and skin aging. Dermatoendocrinol 2012; 4(3): 298–307.

Schleusener J., Salazar A., von Hagen J. et al. Retaining skin barrier function properties of the stratum corneum with components of the natural moisturizing factor — a randomized, placebo-controlled double-blind in vivo study. Molecules 2021; 26(6): 1649.

Schmuth M., Blunder S., Dubrac S. et al. Epidermal barrier in hereditary ichthyoses, atopic dermatitis, and psoriasis. J Dtsch Dermatol Ges 2015; 13(11): 1119–1123.

Schons K.R., Beber A.A., Beck Mde O., Monticielo O.A. Nail involvement in adult patients with plaque-type psoriasis: prevalence and clinical features. An Bras Dermatol 2015; 90(3): 314–319.

Schwartz J., Friedman A.J. Exogenous factors in skin barrier repair. J Drugs Dermatol 2016; 15(11): 1289–1294.

Schwarz A., Bruhs A., Schwarz T. The short-chain fatty acid sodium butyrate functions as a regulator of the skin immune system. J Investig Dermatol 2017; 137(4): 855–864.

Scott I.R. The natural process of skin moisturization. In: The new generation of skin care science, edited by V. Research, pp. 6–10. Morris Plains, NJ: Cosmetic Dermatology, 1993.

Sekhon S., Jeon C., Nakamura M. et al. Review of the mechanism of action of coal tar in psoriasis. J Dermatolog Treat 2018; 29(3): 230–232.

Shin S.M., Itson-Zoske B., Fan F. et al. Peripheral sensory neurons and non-neuronal cells express functional Piezo1 channels. Mol Pain 2023; 19: 17448069231174315.

Sidbury R., Sullivan A.F., Thadhani R.I., Camargo C.A. Jr. Randomized controlled trial of vitamin D supplementation for winter-related atopic dermatitis in Boston: a pilot study. Br J Dermatol 2008; 159(1): 245–247.

Simopoulos A.P. The importance of the omega-6/omega-3 fatty acid ratio in cardiovascular disease and other chronic diseases. Exp Biol Med 2002; 227(6): 409–421.

Siu P.L.K., Choy C.T., Chan H.H.Y. et al. A novel multi-strain E3 probiotic formula improved the gastrointestinal symptoms and quality of life in Chinese psoriasis patients. Microorganisms 2024; 12(1): 208.

Slominski A.T., Li W., Kim T.-K. et al. Novel activities of CYP11A1 and their potential physiological significance. J Steroid Biochem Mol Biol 2015; 151: 25–37.

Smythe P., Wilkinson H.N. The skin microbiome: current landscape and future opportunities. Int J Mol Sci 2023; 24(4): 3950.

Solakoglu Ö., Heydecke G., Amiri N., Anitua E. The use of plasma rich in growth factors (PRGF) in guided tissue regeneration and guided bone regeneration. A review of histological, immunohistochemical, histomorphometrical, radiological and clinical results in humans. Ann Anat 2020; 231: 151528.

Song E.J., Lee J.A., Park J.J. et al. A study on seasonal variation of skin parameters in Korean males. Int J Cosmet Sci 2015; 37(1): 92–97.

Song H., Yoo Y., Hwang J. et al. Faecalibacterium prausnitzii subspecies-level dysbiosis in the human gut microbiome underlying atopic dermatitis. J Allergy Clin Immunol 2016; 137(3): 852–860.

Szabó K., Bolla B.S., Erdei L. et al. Are the cutaneous microbiota a guardian of the skin's physical barrier? The intricate relationship between skin microbes and barrier integrity. Int J Mol Sci 2023; 24(21): 15962.

Szántó M., Dózsa A., Antal D. et al. Targeting the gut–skin axis — Probiotics as new tools for skin disorder management? Exp Dermatol 2019; 28(11): 1210–1218.

Taibjee S.M., Cheung S.T., Laube S., Lanigan S.W. Controlled study of excimer and pulsed dye lasers in the treatment of psoriasis. Br J Dermatol 2005; 153(5): 960–966.

Tammi R., Ripellino J.A., Margolis R.U., Tammi M. Localization of epidermal hyaluronic acid using the hyaluronate binding region of cartilage proteoglycan as a specific probe. J Invest Dermato 1988; 90(3): 412–414.

Tanaka T., Kouda K., Kotani M. et al. Vegetarian diet ameliorates symptoms of atopic dermatitis through reduction of the number of peripheral eosinophils and of PGE2 synthesis by monocytes. J Physiol Anthropol Appl Human Sci 2001; 20(6): 353–361.

Taneja A., Trehan M., Taylor C.R. 308-nm excimer laser for the treatment of psoriasis: induration-based dosimetry. Arch Dermatol 2003; 139(6): 759–764.

Tan-Lim C.S.C., Esteban-Ipac N.A.R., Mantaring J.B.V. et al. Comparative effectiveness of probiotic strains for the treatment of pediatric atopic dermatitis: a systematic review and network meta-analysis. Pediatr Allergy Immunol 2021; 32(1): 124–136.

Tannock G.W., Fuller R., Smith S.L., Hall M.A. Plasmid profiling of members of the family Enterobacteriaceae, Lactobacilli, and Bifidobacteria to study the transmission of bacteria from mother to infant. J Clin Microbiol 1990; 28(6): 1225–1228.

Taylor C.R., Racette A.L. A 308-nm excimer laser for the treatment of scalp psoriasis. Lasers Surg Med 2004; 34(2): 136–140.

Thaçi D., de la Cueva P., Pink A.E. et al. General practice recommendations for the topical treatment of psoriasis: a modified-Delphi approach. BJGP Open 2020; 4(5): bjgpopen20X101108.

Thye A.Y., Bah Y.R., Law J.W. et al. Gut–skin axis: unravelling the connection between the gut microbiome and psoriasis. Biomedicines 2022; 10(5): 1037.

Todberg T., Egeberg A., Zachariae C. et al. Patients with psoriasis have a dysbiotic taxonomic and functional gut microbiota. Br J Dermatol 2022; 187(1): 89–98.

Tokura Y., Hayano S. Subtypes of atopic dermatitis: from phenotype to endotype. Allergol Int 2022; 71(1): 14–24.

Toncic R.J., Jakasa I., Hadzavdic S.L. et al. Altered levels of sphingosine, sphinganine and their ceramides in atopic dermatitis are related to skin barrier function, disease severity and local cytokine milieu. Int J Mol Sci 2020; 13(6): 1958.

Torsekar R., Gautam M.M. Topical therapies in psoriasis. Indian Dermatol Online J 2017; 8(4): 235–245.

Totte J.E., van der Feltz W.T., Hennekam M. et al. Prevalence and odds of Staphylococcus aureus carriage in atopic dermatitis: a systematic review and meta-analysis. Br J Dermatol 2016; 175(4): 687–695.

Uberoi A., Bartow-McKenney C., Zheng Q. et al. Commensal microbiota regulates skin barrier function and repair via signaling through the aryl hydrocarbon receptor. Cell Host Microbe 2021; 29(8): 1235–1248.

Udompataikul M., Huajai S., Chalermchai T. et al. The effects of oral vitamin D supplement on atopic dermatitis: a clinical trial with Staphylococcus aureus colonization determination. J Med Assoc Thail 2015; 98: S23–S30.

Umehara Y., Trujillo-Paez J.V., Yue H. et al. Calcitriol, an active form of vitamin D3, mitigates skin barrier dysfunction in atopic dermatitis NC/Nga mice. Int J Mol Sci 2023; 24(11): 9347.

University of Wisconsin Integrative Health. The Anti-Inflammatory Lifestyle Patient Handout, 2018. https://www.fammed.wisc.edu/files/webfm-uploads/documents/outreach/im/handout_ai_diet_patient.pdf

Valles Y., Artacho A., Pascual-Garcia A. et al. Microbial succession in the gut: directional trends of taxonomic and functional change in a birth cohort of Spanish infants. PLoS Genet 2014; 10(6): e1004406.

Van Cauter E. Diurnal and ultradian rhythms in human endocrine function: a mini-review. Horm Res 1990; 34(2): 45–53.

van Smeden J., Bouwstra J.A. Stratum corneum lipids: their role for the skin barrier function in healthy subjects and atopic dermatitis patients. Curr Probl Dermatol 2016; 49: 8–26.

van Zuuren E.J., Fedorowicz Z., Arents B.W.M. Emollients and moisturizers for eczema: abridged Cochrane systematic review including GRADE assessments. Br J Dermatol 2017; 177(5): 1256–1271.

Vanderwolf K., Kyle C., Davy C. A review of sebum in mammals in relation to skin diseases, skin function, and the skin microbiome. PeerJ 2023; 11: e16680.

Verallo-Rowell V.M., Dillague K.M., Syah-Tjundawan B.S. Novel antibacterial and emollient effects of coconut and virgin olive oils in adult atopic dermatitis. Dermatitis 2008; 19(6): 308–315.

Verdier-Sévrain S., Bonté F. Skin hydration: a review on its molecular mechanisms. J Cosmet Dermatol 2007; 6(2): 75–82.

Vijayashankar M., Raghunath N. Pustular psoriasis responding to probiotics — a new insight. Our Dermatol 2012; 3: 326–329.

Visser M.J.E., Kell D.B., Pretorius E. Bacterial dysbiosis and translocation in psoriasis vulgaris. Front Cell Infect Microbiol 2019; 9: 7.

Voegeli R., Gierschendorf J., Summers B., Rawlings A.V. Facial skin mapping: from single point bio-instrumental evaluation to continuous visualization of skin hydration, barrier function, skin surface pH, and sebum in different ethnic skin types. Int J Cosmet Sci 2019; 41(5): 411–424.

Voegeli R., Rawlings A.V. Corneocare — the role of the stratum corneum and the concept of total barrier care. HPC Today 2013; 8(4): 7–16.

Voegeli R., Rawlings A.V. Moisturizing at a molecular level — the basis of corneocare. Int J Cosmet Sci 2023; 45(2): 133–154.

Volkova N.V., Glazkova L.K., Khomchenko V.V., Sadick N.S. Novel method for rejuvenation using Er:YAG laser equipped with a spatially modulated ablation module: an open prospective uncontrolled cohort study. J Cosmet Laser Ther 2017; 19(1): 25–29.

Voss K.E., Bollag R.J., Fussell N. et al. Abnormal aquaporin-3 protein expression in hyperproliferative skin disorders. Arch Dermatol Res 2011; 303(8): 591–600.

Warner R.R., Myers M.C., Taylor D.A. Electron probe analysis of human skin: determination of the water concentration profile. J Invest Dermatol 1988; 90(2): 218–224.

Watanabe S., Narisawa Y., Arase S. et al. Differences in fecal microflora between patients with atopic dermatitis and healthy control subjects. J Allergy Clin Immunol 2003; 111(3): 587–591.

Watson R.R., Zibadi S., Preedy V.R. Polyphenols in human health and disease. Elsevier Inc., 2014.

Werfel T., Reekers R., Busche M. et al. Association of birch pollen-related food-responsive atopic dermatitis with birch pollen allergen-specific T-cell reactions. Curr Probl Dermatol 1999; 28: 18–28.

Wildnauer R.H., Bothwell J.W., Douglass A.B. Stratum corneum biomechanical properties. I. Influence of relative humidity on normal and extracted human stratum corneum. J Invest Dermatol 1971; 56(1): 72–78.

Wohlrab W. The influence of urea on the penetration kinetics of topically applied corticosteroids. Acta Derm Venereol 1984; 64(3): 233–238.

Wollenberg A., Barbarot S., Bieber T. et al. Consensus-based European guidelines for treatment of atopic eczema (atopic dermatitis) in adults and children: part I. J Eur Acad Dermatol Venereol 2018; 32(5): 657–682.

Wollenberg A., Kinberger M., Arents B. et al. European guideline (EuroGuiDerm) on atopic eczema — part II: non-systemic treatments and treatment recommendations for special AE patient populations. J Eur Acad Dermatol Venereol 2022; 36(110): 1904–1926.

Wollenberg A., Werfel T., Ring J. et al. Atopic dermatitis in children and adults — diagnosis and treatment. Dtsch Arztebl Int 2023; 120(13): 224–234.

Won T.J., Kim B., Lim Y.T. et al. Oral administration of Lactobacillus strains from kimchi inhibits atopic dermatitis in NC/Nga mice. J Appl Microbiol 2011; 110(5): 1195–1202.

Yamada Y., Hasegawa S., Katagiri K. Oral supplementation of hyaluronic acid improves skin hydration: a double-blind, placebo-controlled study. Dermatol Ther 2022; 35(3): e15289.

Yamashiro Y. Probiotics to prebiotics and their clinical use. In: Encyclopedia of Infection and Immunity, edited by N. Rezaei, pp. 674–688. Oxford, UK: Elsevier, 2022.

Yan B.X., Chen X.Y., Ye L.R. et al. Cutaneous and systemic psoriasis: classifications and classification for the distinction. Front Med (Lausanne) 2021; 8: 649408.

Yang L., Mao-Qiang M., Taljebini M. et al. Topical stratum corneum lipids accelerate barrier repair after tape stripping, solvent treatment and some but not all types of detergent treatment. Br J Dermatol 1995; 133(5): 679–685.

Yang S., Zhu T., Wakefield J.S. et al. Link between obesity and atopic dermatitis: does obesity predispose to atopic dermatitis, or vice versa? Exp Dermatol 2023; 32(7): 975–985.

Yen H., Dhana A., Okhovat J.P. et al. Alcohol intake and risk of nonmelanoma skin cancer: a systematic review and dose-response meta-analysis. Br J Dermatol 2017; 177(3): 696–707.

Yokota M., Tokudome Y. The effect of glycation on epidermal lipid content, its metabolism and change in barrier function. Skin Pharmacol Physiol 2016; 29(5): 231–242.

Yokouchi M., Kubo A. Maintenance of tight junction barrier integrity in cell turnover and skin diseases. Exp Dermatol 2018; 27(8): 876–883.

Yokoyama S., Hiramoto K., Koyama M., Ooi K. Impairment of skin barrier function via cholinergic signal transduction in a dextran sulphate sodium-induced colitis mouse model. Exp Dermatol 2015; 24(10): 779–784.

Yosipovitch G., Xiong G.L., Haus E. et al. Time-dependent variations of the skin barrier function in humans: transepidermal water loss, stratum corneum hydration, skin surface pH, and skin temperature. J Invest Dermatol 1998; 110(1): 20–23.

Young M.M., Franken A., du Plessis J.L. Transepidermal water loss, stratum corneum hydration, and skin surface pH of female African and Caucasian nursing students. Skin Res Technol 2019; 25(1): 88–95.

Zaki S.N., Mardyansyah O.C., Purwoko R.Y., Sutanto H.U. Platelet-rich plasma for the treatment of atopic dermatitis: a literature review. J Clin Aesthet Dermatol 2024; 17(7): 43–49.

Zanello S.B., Jackson D.M., Holick M.F. Expression of the circadian clock genes CLOCK and PERIOD1 in human skin. J Invest Dermatol 2000; 115(4): 757–760.

Zaniboni M.C., Samorano L.P., Orfali R.L., Aoki V. Skin barrier in atopic dermatitis: beyond filaggrin. An Bras Dermatol 2016; 91(4): 472–478.

Zelickson B.D., Mehregan D.A., Wendelschfer-Crabb G. et al. Clinical and histologic evaluation of psoriatic plaques treated with a flashlamp pulsed dye laser. J Am Acad Dermatol 1996; 35(1): 64–68.

Zhang J., Loman L., Oldhoff M., Schuttelaar M.L.A. Association between moderate to severe atopic dermatitis and lifestyle factors in the Dutch general population. Clin Exp Dermatol 2022; 47(8): 1523–1535.

Zhang X.E., Zheng P., Ye S.Z. et al. Microbiome: role in inflammatory skin diseases. J Inflamm Res 2024; 17: 1057–1082.

Zheng Y., Hunt R.L., Villaruz A.E. et al. Commensal Staphylococcus epidermidis contributes to skin barrier homeostasis by generating protective ceramides. Cell Host Microbe 2022; 30(3): 301–313.

Zouboulis C.C., Makrantonaki E. Sugar consumption and skin aging. J Derm Res 2022; 45(1): 67–75.

Zuberbier T., Abdul Latiff A., Aggelidis X. et al. A concept for integrated care pathways for atopic dermatitis-A GA^2 LEN ADCARE initiative. Clin Transl Allergy 2023; 13(9): e12299.

www.ingramcontent.com/pod-product-compliance
Lightning Source LLC
Chambersburg PA
CBHW052016030426
42335CB00026B/3166